The Clinical Guide to Oncology Nutrition

Paula Davis McCallum, MS, RD
and Christine Gail Polisena, MS, MBA, RD
Editors

Oncology Nutrition Dietetic Practice Group

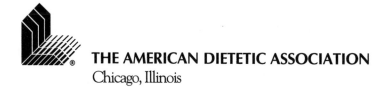

THE AMERICAN DIETETIC ASSOCIATION
Chicago, Illinois

Library of Congress Cataloging-in-Publication Data

The clinical guide to oncology nutrition/Paula Davis McCallum, Christine Gail
Polisena, editors.
     p.; cm.
   Includes bibliographical references and index.
   ISBN 0-88091-177-8 (softbound)
    1. Cancer—Nutritional aspects. 2. Cancer—Diet therapy. I. McCallum, Paula Davis. II.
Polisena, Christine Gail
   [DNLM: 1. Neoplasms—diet therapy. QZ 266 C64147 1999]
   RC271.D52 C57 2000
   616.99'40654—dc21   99-050331

The views expressed in this publication are those of the authors and do not necessarily reflect policies
and/or official positions of The American Dietetic Association. Mention of product names in this publication
does not constitute endorsement by the authors or The American Dietetic Association. The American Dietetic
Association disclaims responsibility for the application of the information contained herein.

10 9 8 7 6 5 4 3 2 1

Contents

Chapter 5
Changes in Carbohydrate, Protein, and Fat Metabolism in Cancer _____53
Linda Nebeling, PhD, MPH, RD

Chapter 6
Chemotherapy and Nutrition Implications _____61
Barbara Eldridge, RD

Chapter 7
Nutrition Concerns with the Radiation Therapy Patient _____70
Christine Gail Polisena, MS, MBA, RD

Chapter 8
Nutrition Implications of Surgical Oncology_____79
Ginny Allison, MS, RD, CNSD; Teresa Dixon, CNSD;
Barbara Eldridge, RD; Rashida Jinnah, MS, RD, CNSD;
Christine Gail Polisena, MS, MBA, RD

Chapter 9
Medical Nutrition Therapy in Bone Marrow Transplantation _____90
Paula M. Charuhas, MS, RD, FADA, CNSD

Chapter 14
Medical Nutrition Therapy in HIV Disease _____134
Cade Fields-Gardner, MS, RD

Chapter 15
Medical Nutrition Therapy in Palliative Care _____143
Anne Cox, MS, RD; Paula Davis McCallum, MS, RD

Chapter 16
Alternative Therapies in Oncology_____150
Laura Molseed, MS, RD

Chapter 17
Nutrition During Cancer Recovery
Daniel W. Nixon, MD

Appendix A
Suggested Management of Nutrition-Related Symptoms
Marnie Dobbin, MS, RD; Virginia W. Hartmuller, PhD, MS, RD, FADA

Appendix B
Common Supportive Drug Therapies Used with Oncology Patients
Leanne D. Kennedy, PharmD

Appendix C
Resources For the Professional and For the Patient
Laura Elliott, RD; Dee Gabbard, RD

Foreword

The Clinical Guide to Oncology Nutrition, authored almost entirely by clinical dietitians, is testimonial to the progressive trend toward effective dietitian specialization in the complex field of neoplastic disease. As emphasized throughout this volume, evaluation of the patient's status early and, if indicated, at suitable intervals provides assurance that nutrition support will be instituted. Forms of support may run the gamut from simple dietary modifications to total parenteral nutrition. For the patient with significant disease and the presence of severe malnutrition or serious risk of developing malnutrition while undergoing anti-tumor treatment, there are, unfortunately, no reliable markers that will predict whether initiation of nutrition support modalities will improve nutritional status. Therefore, efforts at providing appropriate medical nutrition therapy for those at depletion risk are indicated as an integral part of the therapeutic program. As malignancy progresses, its manifestations include a hypercatabolic state with neoplastic syndromes including wasting or cachexia with eventual terminal state despite continuing nutrition support unless reversed by effective anti-tumor therapy. Much has been learned about the various hormones, cytokines, and other peptides released by monocytes, macrophages, and other cells that induce these syndromes. Increased knowledge about these mediators and their modes of action creates the possibility of reversing the hypercatabolic state by inhibiting factors. This, hopefully, would permit better nutrition maintenance of patients in association with more effective anti-tumor modalities.

Dietetics professionals, clinical dietitians, as well as other healthcare professionals, are affected by rapid changes in health care which minimize patient time in hospitals and increase care in outpatient settings, possibly involving surgery, radiation, and/or chemotherapy. How often will the dietetics professional making the initial evaluation be in a position to follow the same patient? How many hospital and outpatient clinical care units include dietitians and have the organization to permit dietitians to be involved with nurses and physicians and other healthcare givers in such settings and with input to home care? These are key questions of care because of the frequent prolonged treatment of such patients. I have the impression that the answers vary greatly from one institution to another and that very much more needs to be done to provide adequate support. The laudatory efforts of the American Dietetic Association, complimented by the very supportive statement of the Institute of Medicine of the National Academy of Science, to have Congress expand coverage of the contributions of clinical dietitians through Medicare should be supported by all professional health groups. A very logical extension of such coverage in the prevention and treatment of cancer is allocation of funds now available to state and local governments from the successful legal suits against the tobacco industry.

Maurice E. Shils, MD, ScD.
Professor Emeritus of Medicine
Cornell University Medical College

Nutrition Consultant Emeritus
Memorial Sloan-Kettering Cancer Center

Preface

The Clinical Guide to Oncology Nutrition was conceived in the early years of the Oncology Nutrition Dietetic Practice Group (ON DPG) of the American Dietetic Association in response to member requests for "practice guidelines." It is intended to be a thorough and accurate reference to be used by dietetics professionals, dietetics interns, medical students and residents, nurses, and other health care professionals. We envision that it will be especially useful to those who cross-cover various areas of oncology, nurses, students, and entry-level dietetics professionals and those who need a ready answer to a "sidewalk consult."

Originally, this publication was intended to be a pocket-sized handbook but during its development, we decided to use a full-size format when it was determined that we had too much material for a pocket-sized book and did not want to eliminate any of the content. *The Clinical Guide to Oncology Nutrition* covers the spectrum of oncology nutrition from prevention to recovery and alternative therapy to palliative care and hospice. There are three appendixes: Symptom Management, Common Supportive Drug Therapies Used in Oncology, and Resources for the Professional and for the Patient and Family. The appendixes contain information that is applicable and referenced throughout the book. Many chapters are cross-referenced to enable easy access to information. Finally, the book features a handy pocket located on the back cover for storage of personal and institution materials, such as formulary cards. Reproducible masters for the Patient-Generated Subjective Global Assessment forms are provided in the pocket.

ON DPG and ADA offer additional publications that integrate well with *The Clinical Guide to Oncology Nutrition. Oncology Nutrition: Patient Education Materials* was developed and published in 1998 in response to member needs. It contains reproducible patient-education materials that can be adapted to meet individual needs in a variety of settings. Guidelines and resources for the professional are also included. The *Patient Education Materials* are referenced several times throughout *The Clinical Guide to Oncology Nutrition. Medical Nutrition Therapy Across the Continuum of Care (MNTACC)* is a publication of the American Dietetic Association in conjunction with Morrison Health Care. Its oncology protocols were developed by ON DPG and are referenced several times in this book.

An instructional video, *Patient-Generated Subjective Global Assessment* (PG-SGA), is currently under development and will soon be available from the American Dietetic Association. The PG-SGA is a quick multidisciplinary tool which can be used in a variety of clinical oncology settings to assess nutrition status and triage medical nutrition therapy. This relatively new nutrition assessment and triage tool is discussed in the second chapter of this book and is also used in *MNTACC.*

Reviewers

Abby S. Bloch, PhD, RD, FADA*
Nutrition Consultant in Private Practice
New York, New York

Nanna Cross, PhD, RD
University of Wyoming Family Practice
Residency Program
Cheyenne, Wyoming

Barbara Eldridge, RD
Clinical Research Associate
University of Colorado Cancer Center
Denver, Colorado

Karen Kulakowski, MA, RD, CNSD*
Oncology Dietitian and WINS Nutritionist
Baystate Health System
Springfield, Massachusetts

Paula Davis McCallum, MS, RD*
Nutrition Consultant
Chagrin Falls, Ohio

Linda Nebeling, PhD, MPH, RD*
Acting Chief—Health Promotion
  Research Branch
Nutritionist—5 A Day Program
National Cancer Institute
Bethesda, Maryland

*Member of Editorial Board

Faith D. Ottery, MD, PhD*
President, Ottery & Associates, Inc.
Director, Clinical Research
Bio-Technology General Corporation
Iselin, NJ

Christine Gail Polisena, MS, MBA, RD
Clinical Dietitian/Wellness Coordinator
Whole Health Management Inc.
Cleveland, Ohio

Declan Walsh, MSc, FACP, FRCP*
Director, Harry R. Horvitz Center for
  Palliative Medicine
Department of Hematology/Medical Oncology
The Taussig Cancer Center
The Cleveland Clinic Foundation
Cleveland, Ohio

Donna L. Weihofen, MS, RD*
Senior Nutritionist
University of Wisconsin Comprehensive
Cancer Center
Madison, Wisconsin

Joyce M. Yasko, PhD, FAAN, RN*
Associate Director, Clinical and Network
  Programs
University of Pittsburgh Cancer Institute
UPMC Health System
Pittsburgh, Pennsylvania

The Oncology Nutrition Dietetic Practice Group of the American Dietetic Association gratefully acknowledges Mead Johnson Nutritionals for providing an educational grant in support of this publication.

Special thanks to Maurice E. Shills, MD, ScD, who wrote the Foreword for this book. Dr. Shills is Professor Emeritus of Medicine, Cornell University Medical College, New York, N.Y. and Nutrition Consultant Emeritus, Memorial Sloan-Kettering Cancer Center, New York, N.Y.

Nutrition and Cancer Prevention

Connie Mobley, PhD, RD

A small percentage of cancers can be explained by genetics. For most people, dietary choices and physical activity are second only to tobacco in determining cancer risk (1). Evolving scientific data support the thesis that all human cancers are likely, to some extent, to be influenced by diet (2). According to Doll and Peto (3), approximately one-third of the 500,000 cancer deaths that occur in the United States yearly are related to dietary factors. Both dietary intake and nutritional status can alter not only the total risk of acquiring a cancer, but also the type of cancer and the age at which it might appear.

Diet and Cancer

Cancer is an assortment of diseases that occur when abnormal cells exhibit uncontrollable growth. The process begins when a procarcinogen has failed to be detoxified or excreted, and is converted to a carcinogen responsible for altering genetic material. Figure 1.1 suggests how dietary factors can act to prevent promotion and progression of mutant cells to latent tumor cells. Other dietary factors act to further promote the carcinogenic process which involves conversion of latent cells to differentiated tumor cells.

Major points to consider when discussing the nutrition and cancer prevention connection include the following:

- The food supply includes hundreds of procarcinogens, cancer promoters, anti-carcinogens, anti-cancer promoters, and cancer inhibitors (4).
- Achieving a balance among all dietary factors, while meeting nutrient needs, is paramount to cancer prevention.
- Cellular integrity and optimum cellular function can bolster the body's ability to detoxify carcinogens by directing the course and outcome of metabolic processes active in the cancer process (5).
- In a natural environment, it is impossible to escape exposure to carcinogenic agents.
- Over time, the aging process and environmental factors can alter cell replication and maintenance. Dietary and endogenous antioxidants are important in maintaining the balance of free radical activity.
- Maintaining health through diet and exercise enhances defense systems and may extend the incubation period of latent cancer cells and the ability of cells to detoxify and inhibit the cancer process.
- Food choices based on principles of variety and moderation, combined with physical activity, can greatly enhance immune system response and the role of homeostasis in maintenance of health.

Figure 1.1   Conceptual overview of the relationship between dietary factors exemplified as possible promoters or inhibitors in carcinogenesis.

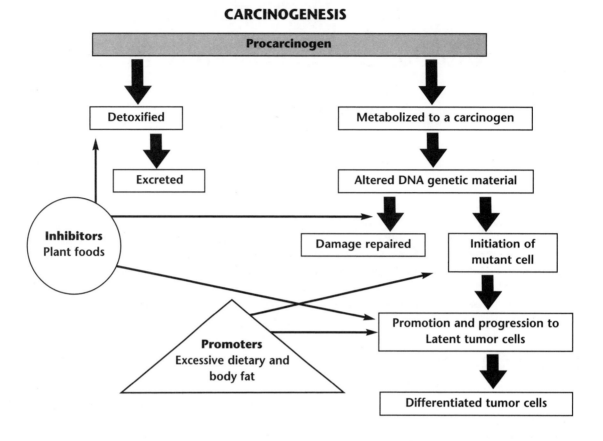

Guidelines on Diet, Nutrition, and Cancer Prevention

The evolution of dietary guidelines for cancer control parallel the development of
- Dietary Guidelines for Americans (6),
- the US Department of Agriculture (USDA) Food Guide Pyramid (7), and
- other initiatives designed to address diet-related conditions associated with chronic disease (8).

    See Table 1.1 for a summary of information included in the 1988 National Cancer Institute (NCI) Dietary Guidelines (9), the 1996 American Cancer Society (ACS) Nutrition Guidelines (10), the Dietary Recommendations of The American Institute for Cancer Research (11), and the USDA Dietary Guidelines (6). Review of contemporary scientific data and the consensus of scientists and health providers precede guideline development. These guidelines can provide direction to dietetics practitioners engaged in cancer prevention strategies.

Plant-based Foods

Epidemiological data strongly support the association between consumption of plant-based foods and reduced risk of cancers of the lung, colon, and rectum (12). Table 1.2 illustrates the potential strength of possible links between diet and site-specific cancers. Plant-based foods contain the essential nutrients that support optimum tissue and organ responses, antioxidants, dietary fibers, and phytochemicals. They act to inhibit cancer by functioning as (13)
- inhibitors of neoplastic transformation by inhibiting hormone-dependent steps in tumor formation and

Table 1.1   Dietary Guidelines and Goals for Cancer Prevention

Agency	Fruits and Vegetables	Dietary Fiber	Dietary Fat	Obesity	Alcohol	Other
American Cancer Society	Choose most foods from plant sources. 5 a day	Choose most foods from plant sources. Breads, cereals, grain products, rice, pasta, or beans several times each day	Limit intake of high-fat foods, particularly those from animal sources. Choose low-fat foods. Limit consumption of meats, especially high-fat meats.	Be physically active. Achieve and maintain a healthy weight. Be at least moderately active for 30 minutes or more on most days of the week.	Limit consumption of alcoholic beverages, if you drink at all.	
National Cancer Institute	Variety 5 a day	20–30 g/day, not to exceed 35 g	Reduce to 30% of calories	Avoid	Consume in moderation, if at all.	Minimize consumption of salt-cured, salt-pickled, and smoked foods.
American Institute for Cancer Research	Choose plant-based diet rich in variety of vegetables, fruits, pulses (legumes), and minimally processed starchy staple foods. Eat 15–30 ounces or >5 servings vegetables and fruits daily.	Eat 20–30 ounces or >7 servings of cereals, legumes, roots, tubers, and plantains daily.	If eaten at all, red meat to provide <10% total energy. Total fats and oils to provide 15% to no more than 30% total energy.	Avoid being over- or underweight and limit weight gain during adulthood to <11 pounds If activity is low or moderate, walk briskly daily for 1 hour and vigorously exercise for 1 hour weekly.	Alcohol not recommended If consumed, limit to <2 drinks/day for men and 1 for women.	Limit salt from all sources to <6 g/day for adults. Store and preserve food properly. Do not eat charred food. Limit refined sugar to <10% total energy daily. For those who follow these goals, dietary supplements are probably unnecessary and possibly unhelpful for reducing cancer risk.
USDA, US Dept. of Health & Human Services	Choose a diet with plenty of grain products, vegetables, and fruits.	Choose a diet with plenty of grain products, vegetables, and fruit.	Choose a diet low in fat, saturated fat, and cholesterol.	Balance the food you eat with physical activity. Maintain or improve your weight. Total fats and oils to provide 15% to no more than 30% total energy.	If you drink alcoholic beverages, do so in moderation.	Eat a variety of foods. Choose a diet moderate in salt and sodium. Choose a diet moderate in sugars.

protecting genetic material from carcinogenic agents;
- suppressers of free radical production;
- bulking agents to dilute carcinogens and decrease gastrointestinal transit time;
- stimulators of physiologically active anti-cancer enzymes.

See Table 1.3 for a list of plant-based foods which are rich in anti-cancer components.

High-fat Diets

Critical experimental research to determine effects of low-fat diets on cancer risk have not been completed. Ecologic studies have identified associations between total fat intake and lung, prostate, colon, breast, endometrium, and ovarian cancers (11,14,15). These associations have been inconclusive and disputed by some. Nonetheless, dietary fat likely stimulates cancer growth and acts as a cancer promoter,

Table 1.2   Association Between Specific Diet and Nutrition Variables and Cancer Sites

Variables	Lung	Rectum Colon	Breast	Prostate	Head and Neck	Kidney and Liver	Endometrial
Plant-based foods, especially fruits and vegetables ↓ Risk	Strong	Strong	Possible	Possible	Probable		Possible
Exercise ↓ Risk		Probable	Possible	Probable			
High fat foods, especially from animal sources ↑ Risk	Possible	Possible	Weak	Probable			Weak
Obesity ↑ Risk		Possible	Possible	Possible		Possible	Strong
Alcohol ↑ Risk		Weak	Possible		Possible		

Key: ● Strong   ◗ Probable   ◖ Possible   ◔ Weak

Table 1.3   Common Plant-based Foods, Anticancer Constituents, and Their Roles in Cancer Prevention

Food	Pytochemical	Vitamin	Fiber	Antioxidant Activity	Stimulates Anticancer Enzymes	Acts as a Cancer Inhibitor
Garlic, onion (Allium vegetable)	Organosulfur compounds					
Broccoli, cauliflower, cabbage, and other cruciferous vegetables (Brassica vegetable)	Indoles Sulforaphane Isothiocynate	Folate Vitamin A Vitamin C	Insoluble			X
Citrus fruit	Terpenes Coumarins Flavonoids	Vitamin C Folate	Soluble	X	X	X
Strawberries, grapes, apples, berries, and nuts	Ellagic acid	Vitamin E Vitamin C Beta Carotene	Soluble	X	X	X
Carrots, yams, cantaloupe, butternut squash		Beta Carotene	Soluble Insoluble	X	X	X
Soybeans, beans, peas, lentils	Genistein (other isoflavones) Saponins Phytosterols		Soluble			X
Hot peppers	Capsaicin	Vitamin C		X		X
Flaxseed, wheat, barley, whole wheat, brown rice	Lignans		Soluble Insoluble	X		X
Tomatoes, red grapefruit	Lycopene	Vitamin C	Soluble	X		
Green tea, grapes	Polyphenols					X

after initial mutagenic steps have taken place. It also may be a mutagen through oxidation of fatty acids and production of free radicals that damage genetic material. Studies-in-progress continue to examine the following (15,16,17):

- total fat intake related to obesity, percent body fat, body fat distribution, and sex-hormone levels
- dietary fat intake related to intake of fat-soluble carcinogens, especially animal fat
- dietary fat intake related to fruit and vegetable intake
- other nutrient components in modifying the role of dietary fat intake
- type of dietary fat (saturated, n-6-polyunsaturated, n-3-fats) on mechanisms of cancer progression
- the role of short-chain fatty acids in the carcinogenic process

Body Weight and Physical Activity

It has been hypothesized that obesity and associated inactivity are major determinants of colon and sex hormone–related cancers like prostate, breast, edometrial, and ovarian cancer. Whether it is total fat in the diet or the increased body mass associated with obesity that increases risk for cancer is a continuing debate.

Total energy intake is strongly associated with breast cancer in postmenopausal women, and physical activity may have a protective effect in promoting energy balance and preventing weight gain. Yet heavier women appear to be at decreased risk for developing premenopausal cancer (18). It appears that adverse patterns of weight management throughout the life cycle may contribute to increased risk for cancer (19). Obesity and weight gain (which on average is about 10 lb total or 1 lb per year between perimenopause and postmenopause) appear to be related to breast cancer risk (18). Higher serum estrogen levels in obese women, secondary to a high fat intake, is related to increased risk for breast cancer (15). Studies suggest that avoiding weight gain and accumulation of central body fat during adult life may reduce risk of both endometrial and postmenopausal breast cancer (20).

Women and men with lifelong participation in sports activities, and particularly women who spent an average of 3.8 hours per week in physical activities, had lower risk of colon and reproductive cancers (2,21). Levels of prostaglandins, mediated by increased physical activity and a direct effect of activity on decreased transit time in the colon, may be effective in slowing progression of colon cancer. However, exhausting exercise may have an opposite effect (2).

Some have speculated that it is the association between increased physical activity and improved dietary intake that may decrease risk for cancer. Animal studies have shown that energy restriction enhances repair of genetic material (22). The effect occurs when these animals either restrict energy intake or increase energy output to create energy deficits that lead to weight loss.

Other Dietary Issues

Alcohol Intake

Risk of squamous cell carcinoma of the head and neck anatomy has consistently been related to all types of alcohol consumed. Possible relationships between alcohol intake and colon, stomach, pancreatic, liver, and breast cancer have also been identified. Alcohol may be contaminated with carcinogens like N-Nitroso compounds (micotoxins, urethane), inorganic arsenic, and asbestos; it can also act as a solvent for other carcinogens. Additionally, those who consume excessive alcohol may displace micronutrients such as folate and vitamins C and E, which have been associated with decreased cancer risk (23). Nonetheless, moderate alcohol intake may decrease risk of other chronic diseases, such as cardiovascular disease (6).

Food Safety

The food supply contains numerous naturally occurring carcinogens. Therefore, it is impossible to eat a carcinogenic-free diet. Aflatoxins in peanuts, safrol in some plant oils, tannins in grains and grapes, and benzo(a)pyrene formed by smoking meat and fish are just some examples (24). Additionally, potential carcinogens exist as natural metabolites of plant foods like celery, parsley, figs, mustard, pepper, and citrus oils. These products are speculated to be part of the plant's natural defense system. However, laboratory data indicate potential risk only when these natural metabolites are consumed in highly concentrated amounts, well beyond typical dietary consumption. Thus, ingestion of these naturally occurring potential carcinogens is very low. If fruits and vegetables are properly handled and stored, there is no evidence to suggest that they cause any adverse health effects (11). However, naturally found compounds in plants exceed the limits set by the federal government for intake of synthetic carcinogens, such as pesticides and other additives, by a factor of at least 10,000 (24). Federal regulatory agencies assure safe levels of these substances, and some additives, like BHA and BHT, may even have a protective effect against cancer. Yet due to limitations of assessing such minute substances in the diet, there are no relevant epidemiological data to support this premise (11). Concern about either naturally occurring or synthetic carcinogens in the food supply can be addressed by

- choosing in-season, locally grown produce;
- rinsing fruits and vegetables and removing outer leaves before eating;
- practicing food storage and preparation techniques to preserve optimum nutritional value (proper food storage temperatures can delay growth of potent fungal carcinogens);
- marinating protein foods to decrease total cooking time;
- using cooking methods to avoid contact of foods and food drippings with flames;
- using lower cooking temperatures to control occurrence of carcinogens, like the hetrocyclic amines, which are formed when protein foods are broiled.

Questionable Dietary Approaches to Cancer Prevention

Products and Regimens

Dietary and herbal supplements

Nutrient, fiber, phytochemical, and more recently, herbal supplementation are controversial in nature. Until recently, there were few documented scientific trials to test the efficacy of their use. Unfortunately, some of these trials have demonstrated negative findings which do not support use of single high dose supplementation in select high risk groups such as smokers or heavy alcohol consumers. The 1994 Alpha-tocopherol and Beta-carotene (ATBC) study in 29,133 Finnish male smokers showed increased lung cancer and mortality with a supplementation protocol of 20 mg ß-carotene and 50 mg of vitamin E daily. The Beta Carotene and Retinol Efficacy Trial (CARET) conducted in the US was halted due to similar trends in negative results (25). The CARET randomized intervention trial included 18,312 male subjects who smoked > 5 cigarettes per day and received a similar supplementation regimen as the Finnish subjects. By contrast, several small clinical intervention studies have shown a positive response of precancerous oral lesions to 30 mg ß-carotene daily (26). These data indicate that dietary components in supplement form may have possible benefit or possible harm depending upon the type of cancer and potential role the nutrient plays in genetic repair processes. Further research is needed.

The increasing popularity of alternative medicine has stimulated wide interest in the use of herbs as cancer preventives. Those herbal and plant derivatives shown to be effective anticancer agents, like catharanthus, podophyllum, and Pacific yew (family Texaceae), are available by prescription only. Others, like pau d'arco and mistletoe, are unproven anticancer agents and may be harmful (27). Individuals choosing herbal therapeutics and supplementation should be informed of possible negative consequences and encouraged to explore possible alternatives, including a diet based on variety and moderation. Health care professionals should investigate new products and claims, and remain well informed. Further information can be found in the chapter on alternative therapies (see Chapter 16, *Alternative Therapies in Oncology*).

Elimination and restricted dietary regimens

Of the various dietary regimens touted to support cancer prevention, the macrobiotic diet is the most common. Based primarily on whole grains, vegetables, beans, and lentils, it excludes major sources of essential nutrients. Fish, nuts, and fruit are included only occasionally, and dairy and animal products are excluded. This diet has not demonstrated efficacy in cancer control and may increase risk for nutritional deficits that include protein, calcium, and other micronutrients (28). Dietary selections based on variety and moderation are more likely to provide the multitude of anti-cancer agents available in the food supply and contribute to the dilution of cancer promoting agents.

Guidelines for Critiquing New Products and Diets

The following questions should be explored in determining the efficacy of a product or diet in cancer control.

- Does an expert body of reputable nutrition experts or scientists support the efficacy of the product or diet? Anecdotal information cannot replace controlled studies. The National Center for Complementary and Alternative Medicine and the National Cancer Institute at the National Institutes of Health can provide current information about products being tested in clinical trials. Check their web sites in Appendix D for the most current up-to-date information.
- Is there documented evidence that this product or diet is safe? The number who participated in trials and testing is important to note. The word of only a few, or the lack of clinical trial evidence, should be viewed with reservation.
- Does this diet recommend elimination of certain foods or nutrients? If so, what is the rationale? Balance and variety are designed to enhance the synergy of food constituents to promote health. The stress involved in following a restricted diet can be a health risk factor.
- Does the product make singular unfounded claims? A product may act as an antioxidant, yet still produce toxic by-products or imbalances when consumed in large concentrated quantities.
- Is the cost of the product or diet excessive in comparison to a well-balanced diet?
- Does the product appear to be harmless? If so, even the placebo effect can have positive consequences that cannot be ignored, and the practice should not be necessarily discouraged.

Promoting Dietary Guidelines

Keep the Message Simple

Decreasing cancer risk and promoting cancer control hinge on positive dietary behavior changes. Health care professionals need to follow a few simple rules and use the simplest, most familiar tools in conveying the message:

- Base dietary recommendations on the Food Guide Pyramid (Figure 1.2).
- Determine the client's orientation in the stages of change model (Box 1.1) (29).
- Focus on only one message at a time. Provide guidance and information to meet the specific needs and desires of the client. Remind client that behavioral change is a multi-step process that takes extended time to accomplish.
- Communicate with other health care providers to seek reinforcement of the nutrition message with your client.

Box 1.1   Stages of Change Model

Precontemplation	Client is unaware that change is necessary. Client is resistant to modifying behavior.
Contemplation	Client is aware and is considering action; no commitment to change
Preparation	Client is ready to change in next 30 days. Some preliminary action is taken
Action	Client makes effort to change a targeted behavior.
Maintenance	Behavior change is stabilized. Relapse is not likely for extended time

Figure 1.2   A Food Guide Pyramid Designed for Nutrition Education and Cancer Prevention

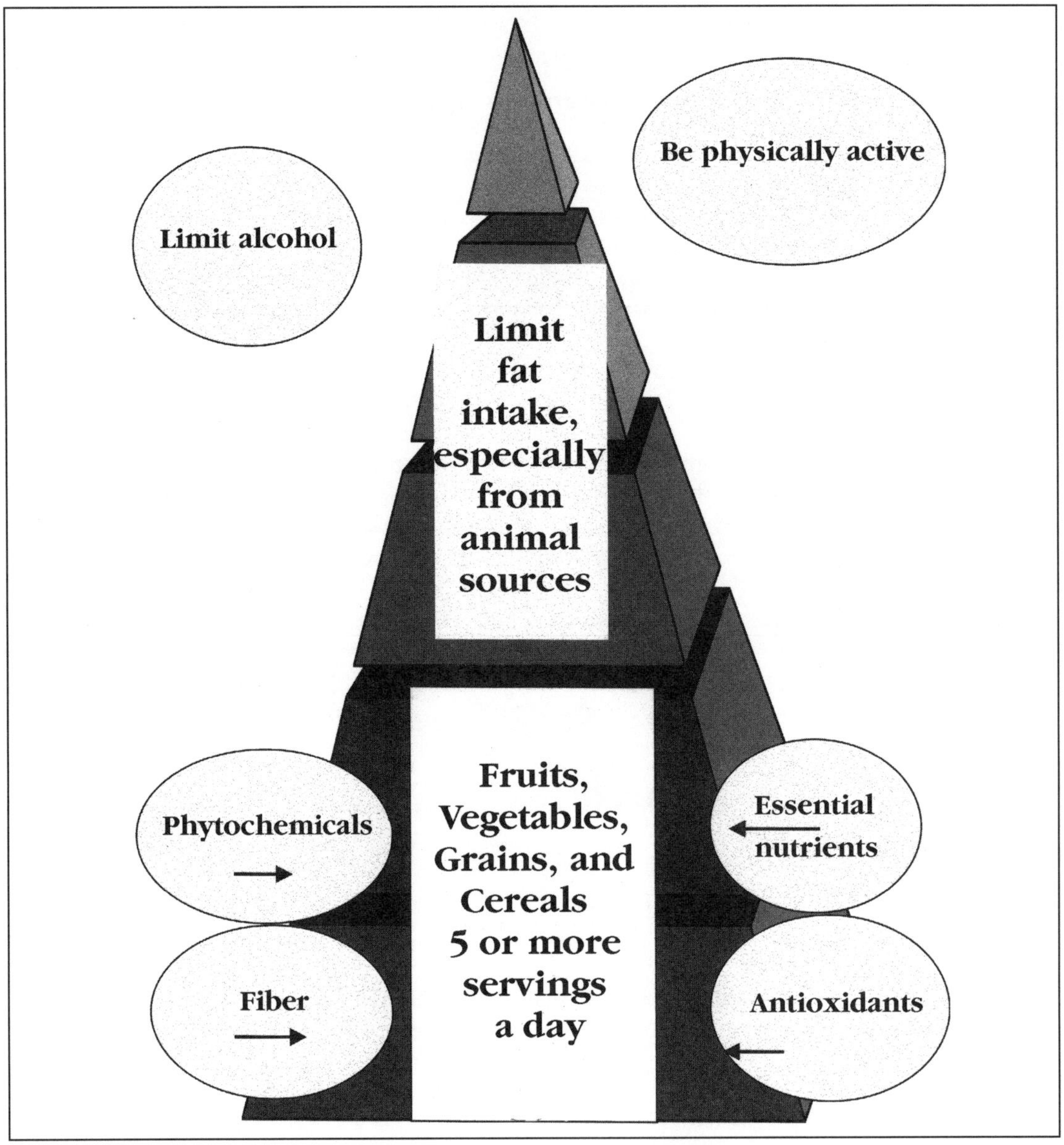

Reprinted with permission from the U.S. Department of Agriculture.

Summary

The scientific evidence that relates diet and nutrition to cancer risk in human populations suggests that diet and physical activity patterns can modify risk of cancer at all stages of its development. Dietary guidelines for cancer control promote plant-based and low-fat foods. A balance of caloric intake and physical activity to promote weight management may also have a positive additive effect on risk. Associations between site-specific cancers and dietary variables such as alcohol intake and food safety may be addressed by promoting food consumption, selection, preparation, and storage practices that promote good nutrition and simultaneously diminish cancer risk. Additionally, questionable dietary practices and products such as botanicals and herbs should be discouraged. Instead, guidelines for critiquing new products and diets should be included in diet and cancer-risk-reduction education initiatives. Finally, messages to promote diet and cancer control should be tailored to address individual needs and concerns and ultimately focus on reinforcing nutrition and diet to promote health.

References

1. McGinnis JM, Foege WH. Actual causes of death in the United States. *JAMA*. 1993;270:2207-2212.
2. Thorling EB. Obesity, fat intake, energy balance, exercise and cancer risk a review. *Nutr Res*. 1996;16(2):315-368.
3. Doll R, Peto R. The causes of cancer: quantitative estimates of avoidable risks of cancer in the United States today. *J Natl Cancer Inst*. 1981;66:1191-1308.
4. Ames BN, Gold LS, Willett WC. The causes and prevention of cancer. *Proc Natl Acad Sci USA*. 1995;92:5258-5265.
5. Boutwell RK. Nutrition and carcinogensis: historical highlights and future prospects. In: Longnecker JB, Kritchevsky D, Drezner MK, eds. *Nutrition and Biotechnology in Heart Disease and Cancer*. New York, NY: Plenum Press; 1995:111-123.
6. *Nutrition and Your Health: Dietary Guidelines for Americans*. 4th ed. Washington, DC: US Depts of Agriculture and Health and Human Services; 1995. Home and Garden Bulletin No. 232.
7. *The Food Guide Pyramid. A Guide To Daily Food Choices*. Washington, DC: US Dept of Agriculture, Human Nutrition Information Services; 1992. Home and Garden Bulletin No. 252.
8. *Healthy People 2000: National Health Promotion and Disease Prevention Objectives*. Washington, DC: US Dept of Health and Human Services; 1990. DHHS (PHS) publication 91-50212.
9. Butrum RR, Clifford CK, Lanza E. NCI dietary guidelines: rationale. *Am J Clin Nutr*. 1988;48:888-895.
10. The American Cancer Society 1996 Advisory Committee on Diet, Nutrition, and Cancer Prevention. Guidelines on diet, nutrition, and cancer prevention: reducing the risk of cancer with healthy food choices and physical activity. *CA Cancer J Clin*. 1996;46:325-341.
11. World Cancer Research Fund in Association with American Institute for Cancer Research. *Food, Nutrition and the Prevention of Cancer: a Global Perspective*. Washington, DC: American Institute for Cancer Research; 1997.
12. Steinmetz KA, Potter JD. Vegetables, fruit, and cancer. I. Epidemiology. *Cancer Causes Control*. 1991;2:325-356.
13. Steinmetz KA, Potter JD. Vegetables, fruit, and cancer. II. Mechanisms. *Cancer Causes Control*. 1991;2:427-442.
14. Greenwald P. The potential of dietary modification to prevent cancer. *Prev Med*. 1996;25:41-43.
15. Kuller LH. Dietary fat and chronic diseases: epidemiologic overview. *J Am Diet Assoc*. 1997;97(suppl):S9-S15.
16. Weisburger JH. Dietary fat and risk of chronic disease: mechanistic insights from experimental studies. *J Am Diet Assoc*. 1997;97(suppl):S16-S23.
17. Greenwald P, Sherwood K, McDonald SS. Fat, caloric intake, and obesity: lifestyle risk factors for breast cancer. *J Am Diet Assoc*. 1997;97(suppl):S24-S30.
18. Hunter DJ, Willett WC. Nutrition and breast cancer. *Cancer Causes Control*. 1996;7:56-68.
19. Ziegler RG. Anthropometry and breast cancer. *J Nutr*. 1997;125(55);924S-928S.
20. Ballard-Barbash R, Swanson CA. Body weight: estimation of risk for breast and endometrial cancers. *Am J Clin Nutr*. 1996;63(suppl):437S-441S.
21. Bernstein L, Henderson BE, Hanisch R, Sullivan-Halley J, Ross RK. Physical exercise and reduced risk of breast cancer in young women. *J Natl Cancer Inst*. 1994;86:1403-1408.
22. Kritchevsky D. The effect of over- and undernutrition on cancer. *Eur J Cancer Prev*. 1995;4(6):445-451.
23. Rothman KJ. Research and prevention priorities for alcohol carcinogenesis. *Environ Health Perspect*. 1995;103(58):161-163.
24. Sugimura T, Wakabayashi K. Carcinogens in foods. In: Shils ME, Olson JA, Skile M, Ross AC, eds. *Modern Nutrition in Health and Disease*. 9th ed. Philadelphia, Pa: Lea and Fibiger; 1999:1255-1261.
25. Rowe PM. Beta-carotene takes a collective beating. *Lancet*. 1996;347:249.
26. Albanes D, Hartman TJ. Antioxidants and cancer: evidence from human observational studies and intervention trials. In: Papas M, ed. *Antioxidant Status, Diet, Nutrition, and Health*. Boca Raton, Fla: CRC Press Inc; 1999:497-544.
27. Robbins EJ, Tyler VE. *Tyler's Herb of Choice: The Therapeutic Use of 24*. 2nd ed. New York, NY: Pharmaceutical Products Press; 1998.

28. Barrett S, Jarvis WT, eds. *The Health Robbers.* Buffalo, NY: Prometheus Books; 1993.

29. Sigman-Grant M. Stages of change: a framework for nutrition interventions. *Nutr Today.* 1996;31(4):162–170.

30. Wang H, Guohua C, Prior RL. Total antioxidant capacity of fruits. *J Agric Food Chem.* 1996;44:701–705.

2

Patient-Generated Subjective Global Assessment

Paula Davis McCallum, MS, RD

Today, traditional hospital settings provide care for more acutely ill patients with shorter lengths of stay than 10 years ago. There have been shifts in health care delivery from traditional inpatient settings to outpatient clinics and alternative sites of health care. Dietetics professionals must identify and care for cancer patients in this new arena, often with fewer human resources than ever before. The Joint Commission on Accreditation of Healthcare Organizations (JCAHO) has recognized nutrition as an important component of patient outcomes. In the inpatient setting, nutrition screening is required within 24 hours of admission (1). Additionally, it is required that the nutrition care process (screening, assessment, and intervention) be interdisciplinary in scope. Similar requirements have recently been included for homecare and hospice (2).

Aggressive identification and treatment of nutrition-related symptoms can stabilize or reverse weight loss in 50% to 88% of oncology cases (3). The Subjective Global Assessment (SGA) of nutrition status is a validated nutrition assessment tool that is appropriate for use in alternative sites, as well as traditional health care settings (4–6). Modifications have been made to the SGA with the Patient-Generated Subjective Global Assessment (PG-SGA) and subsequent Scored PG-SGA. The newest generation of SGA, the Scored PG-SGA is here discussed as a method that is widely applicable in our changing health care environment.

Traditional Nutrition Assessment

Traditional nutrition screening and assessment includes objective measures, such as indices of visceral protein stores, delayed hypersensitivity skin testing (DHST), and anthropometry. These parameters may be altered by a number of conditions including, but not limited to, age, changes in hydration, or immunosuppression. In today's health care arena, laboratory testing is kept to a minimum. Indices of visceral protein stores are infrequently ordered in an alternative setting or during a short hospitalization, based on the premise that such tests increase cost and offer questionable benefit to patient care.

Subjective Global Assessment

In contrast to traditional methods of nutrition assessment, the SGA allows a global assessment of the patient's nutrition status based on a nutrition-related history and physical examination. This assessment does not include laboratory tests, skinfold measurements, or DHST. The SGA was developed at the University of Toronto and the Toronto General Hospital (7). This nutrition assessment instrument has shown superior sensitivity and specificity as a nutrition assessment tool to albumin, transferrin, DHST, anthropometry, creatinine-height index, and the prognostic nutrition index (5). Additionally, the SGA is easy to teach and has a high degree of inter-rater agreement (5). The SGA can be used to predict who needs nutrition intervention and who will benefit from intense nutrition support (8).

The patient history components of the SGA include sections on weight loss, dietary intake, presence of nutrition impact symptoms, functional capacity, and the metabolic demands of the underlying disease. The physical examination considers loss of subcutaneous fat and presence of muscle wasting, edema, or ascites. Each category is rated as mild, moderate or severe. Based on the overall assessment, the patient is assigned an SGA rating of A = well nourished, B = moderately malnourished or at risk for developing malnutrition, or C = severely malnourished. An improvement in nutrition status, even in patients who appear to be severely malnourished, merits a rating of A on subsequent SGAs. The rating of A, B, or C is based on a global assessment including both historical (weight, intake, nutrition impact symptoms, and functional capacity) and physical examination (see Figure 2.2, Table 5). The historical component is weighted slightly more than the physical (60% and 40%, respectively). Ratings of A or C (physiologically well nourished versus severely malnourished) are more straightforward with the predominance of parameters falling in the A or C columns, respectively. The B rating is more ambiguous and may include parameters in any or all columns (remembering that the historical aspects have greater impact on the determination of stage of nutrition status). The PG-SGA was developed by Ottery as a modification of the original SGA (9). Additional information concerning oncology symptom assessment is included in the PG-SGA beyond that of the original SGA.

The most time-consuming aspect of the SGA for the clinician is completing the history section with the patient. Rather than have the health care professional act as the rater for the entire SGA, the PG-SGA requires the patient to complete the four history sections. The use of the patient-generated format streamlines nutrition assessment in the clinical oncology setting and involves the patient directly. This allows the clinician to spend the limited time available addressing the problems identified rather than gathering data.

The PG-SGA can be used in both inpatient and outpatient settings. The latter can include the oncology office or clinic, homecare, and hospice, as well as extended care facilities. The use of the same tool in all settings provides a consistent means of identifying patients with malnutrition and measuring outcomes of nutrition intervention as patients move through the spectrum of health care delivery systems. Additionally, there is greater clinician recognition of treatable malnutrition when using the PG-SGA as a screening tool (10).

Scored PG-SGA

The Scored PG-SGA is a further adaptation of the PG-SGA and allows for triaging of specific nutrition interventions, as well as facilitating quantitative outcomes data collection. In addition to the ratings of A, B, or C, there is a numerical score. The numerical score is based on data collected from the PG-SGA up to and including the physical exam. The numerical score provides clinicians with clearer guidelines as to the level of medical nutrition therapy needed in a given case (see Chapter 3, *Medical Nutrition Therapy Protocols*), while the A, B, or C rating provides an overall picture of a patient's current nutriture. Figure 2.1 presents the Scored PG-SGA, which includes the four patient-generated historical components (weight loss, intake, nutrition impact symptoms, and functional capacity), the clinician portion (diagnosis, age, metabolic stress, and physical exam), the global assessment (A = well nourished, B = moderately malnourished or at risk for malnutrition, C = severely malnourished), the total numerical score, and nutritional triage recommendations. Figure 2.2, Tables and Worksheets for PG-SGA Scoring, is used to facilitate data collection and scoring. Detailed instructions on scoring follow in the PG-SGA Scoring Guide section of this chapter. Additionally, an instructional video, *Patient-Generated Subjective Global Assessment*, will soon be available through The Oncology Nutrition Dietetic Practice Group (ON DPG) of The American Dietetic Association (ADA). The video reviews the components of the Scored PG-SGA and depicts the physical exam, reviewing data collection, and scoring. It includes four case studies and twenty self-assessment questions for two continuing-education credits.

The Nutrition-related Physical Examination

History and physical examination are considered to be the cornerstones of patient diagnosis. Unfortunately, the nutritional aspects of the physical examination (with the exception of the obvious cases of obesity and cachexia) are often overlooked or underappreciated, due to lack of clinician education. While physicians and nurses routinely include physical examination as a part of their overall patient assessment, they often are inadequately taught to consider the physical examination from a nutritional perspective. Dietetics professionals may be able to identify the physical findings from a nutritional deficiency, but do not routinely include physical examination as part of their nutrition assessment. The following section includes written guidelines for performing a nutrition-related physical exam.

Global Aspects of Physical Examination

It is important, whenever possible, that the patient wear a hospital gown during examination. Just as overweight patients are able to mask the appearance of excessive weight by their mode of dress, so can patients who have lost significant weight disguise their weight loss.

The observable aspects of general body composition include an assessment of muscle and fat stores, as well as fluid status (see Figure 2.2, Table 4, for a condensed guide to assessment of fat, muscle and fluid status). Under- and overnutrition are best assessed in terms of adipose (subcutaneous fat) stores and then in terms of muscle mass and function.

Assessment of Subcutaneous Fat

The presence of significant fat loss should be assessed by observation of the usual areas where adipose tissue is normally present. One area of particular interest is the fat pads under the eye. Patients with fat loss will have a characteristic hollow eye. Another area of note is the fat pad over the triceps (ie, the back of the upper arm). A fold of skin is pinched to see whether any (and how much) adipose tissue is present between the finger and thumb. And finally, the anterior lower ribs is another site where adipose stores may be examined. The ribs will be apparent in patients with fat loss. Obvious loss of adipose tissue indicates severe energy deficit. The assessment of adipose tissue loss may not be obvious in the obese patient and must be considered in the context of history (eg, a morbidly obese ovarian cancer patient with a recent 60-pound weight loss).

Assessment of Muscle Mass

Assessment of muscle must include consideration of muscle volume (compared with normal composition), muscle tone, functionality, and gender. In general, the muscles of the upper body are more susceptible to muscle loss during nutritional deprivation, independent of the patient's functional status. However, muscle loss from inactivity and/or bed rest is most prominent in the muscles of the pelvis and upper leg. Areas of assessment for muscle loss include the observation of hollowing of the temples (wasting of the temporalis), prominence of the clavicle (loss of pectoral and deltoids), squaring of the shoulders (loss of deltoids), flattening of the interosseous muscles in the area between the thumb and forefinger, prominence of the scapula (loss of latissimus dorsi, trapezius, and deltoids), and loss of muscle mass of the thigh (quadriceps) or calf (gastrocnemius).

Assessment of Fluid Status

The malnourished cancer patient may be taking inadequate fluids in conjunction with inadequate nutrition, adequate fluid in the face of low calorie and/or protein intake, or receiving supplemental hydration intravenously, as with chemotherapy.

Fluid status is important to the assessment in terms of the 1) hydration of the patient (euvolemic, overhydrated, or dehydrated), 2) the oncotic status as determined by the patient's total body and serum protein status, and 3) abnormal fluid accumulations due to organic or mechanical abnormalities. The two components of fluid status that need to be assessed include tissue turgor and presence of ascites. Tissue turgor can either be decreased as in dehydration or increased (increased firmness, with or without the presence of edema). Decreased tissue turgor seen in dehydration may be associated with skin "tenting." This is assessed by gently pinching a fold of skin. In normal hydration, the skin will spring back into place when the pinched skin is released. In marked dehydration, however, the skin will only slowly return to its normal position. Increased tissue turgor is generally identified as edema. It can be present in a number of conditions including malnutrition with hypoalbuminema, renal or cardiac failure, decreased venous or lymphatic return from the distal aspect of the upper or lower extremities. Edema assessment is best carried out by observing the dependent areas of the body (ie, the ankle and/or sacrum [tail bone]). In the ambulatory patient, the ankle is most commonly involved (pedal edema) and easy to assess by noting impressions left in the skin after gently squeezing the top of the foot, ankle, and/or front of the lower leg. It is important to note that the presacral edema is more common in patients who are bed-bound or sitting through most of the day. In the bed-bound, euvolemic, hypoalbuminemic patient, sacral edema can be marked with little or no pedal edema present.

Ascites (accumulation of fluid in the abdominal cavity) may be present in a number of conditions including malnutrition, liver failure, and intra-abdominal carcinomatosis. Presence of ascites in patients undergoing peritoneal dialysis is difficult to appreciate. The presence of ascites in some patients, such as those with carcinomatosis, may be multifactorial in etiology. The ascites may be related to either excessive peritoneal fluid production or impaired absorption due to impaired lymphatic drainage. The drainage of ascitic fluid through repeat paracentesis is important in the context of nutrition assessment in that it can further contribute to the protein requirements of the patient who is already at risk for malnutrition.

PG-SGA Scoring Guide (10)

Rationale for Scoring

Cooperative oncology groups use toxicity scales throughout their protocols to evaluate patients' tolerance to various anti-neoplastic treatments. These toxicity scales generally use a point system from grade 0 to 4, based on increasing levels of toxicity. Grades 0 through 2 include toxicities that are expected and/or tolerated. Grade 3 toxicities are considered severe and generally indicate the need for some type of intervention, such as a dose modification or treatment delay. Grade 4 toxicity is defined as life-threatening.

With these toxicity scales in mind, a similar system was developed for scoring screening parameters used in the PG-SGA in terms of increasing impact on nutritional status or risk. Moreover, scoring of the PG-SGA goes one step further by providing guidelines for the triage of medical nutrition therapy in addition to a rating for the global assessment of patients' nutriture (11,12). (See Chapter 3, *Medical Nutrition Therapy Protocols*.) Points are assigned to individual segments of the PG-SGA depending on the impact made on nutrition status:

    0 points = minimal impact on nutritional status or risk for deficit
    1 point = mild impact
    2 points = moderate impact
    3 points = potentially severe impact
    4 points = potentially life-threatening

Numeric Scoring versus Subjective *A, B, C* Global Ratings

The scoring technique does not replace the importance of the subjective global assessment of *A, B,* or *C,* as previously defined. The subjective global assessment rating is just that, the clinician's assessment of the patient's nutrition status at a given time. The numeric score allows for initiation of the appropriate pathways for medical nutrition therapy. In many settings, it may be effective to assign a nurse, physician's assistant or other health care professional to score the PG-SGA and refer individual cases to a dietetics professional when appropriate (see Triage for Medical Nutrition Therapy below and Chapter 3, *Medical Nutrition Therapy Protocols*). The triage of medical nutrition therapy based on the numeric scoring of the PG-SGA is a quick multidisciplinary approach which allows for identification and treatment of patients with malnutrition (and those who are at risk for developing malnutrition) in a variety of oncology care venues. The specific instructions for scoring each section of the PG-SGA follow.

Scoring Weight Loss (Figure 2.2, Table 1)

The weight loss scoring is based on the prognostic data of Blackburn et al (13). Patients were noted to have a statistically increased risk of morbidity and mortality when weight loss was greater than 2% per week, greater than 5% per month, greater than 7.5% in 3 months and greater than 10% in 6 months. Weight loss is therefore graded as severe (3 points) if loss is $\geq$ 5% at 1 month or $\geq$ 10% at 6 months. Life threatening is empirically defined to be twice that.

The scoring of weight loss is determined by adding subacute and acute weight changes. Subacute weight loss is based on weight loss during the previous one-month period. *Only if that information is unavailable* is the weight loss for the previous 6-month period used. *The two are not additive* for the overall scoring of the PG-SGA.

Point scores for acute weight loss during the past 2 weeks is found in parentheses directly next to the patient responses on the PG-SGA form (Figure 2.1). *These points (weight loss in past 2 weeks and weight loss over past months [or past 6 months if past (one)-month weight is not available]) are additive and make up the total score for the weight loss section.* The score is recorded in the corresponding box provided in Figure 2.1 and Figure 2.2, Table 1.

Scoring of Food Intake

The score for this section is not additive. The box (Figure 2.1) checked with the highest point value in parentheses is the total score for the section and is to be recorded in the corresponding box in Figure 2.1.

Scoring of Nutrition Impact Symptoms

This section is additive. Add the points given for each symptom checked (Figure 2.1). The total is the score for this section and is to be recorded in the corresponding box in Figure 2.1.

Scoring of Activities and Functions

The score for this section is not additive. The box checked (Figure 2.1) with the highest point value in parentheses is the total score for the section and is to be recorded in the corresponding box in Figure 2.1.

Scoring of Clinician Section of the PG-SGA

The scoring criteria for diseases and/or conditions are found in Figure 2.2, Table 2. *The score is additive for this section* and is recorded in box B on both sides of the PG-SGA form (Figures 2.1 and 2.2).

The scoring system for metabolic stress factors is found in Figure 2.2, Table 3. Points are accumulated for presence of fever *or* fever duration, whichever is greater, *but not both.* Additional points are accumulated for chronic steroid use as shown in Figure 2.2, Table 3. Fever score is added to steroid score such that a patient having a fever of > 102 degrees for < 72 hours (3 points, based on the higher score for presence of fever, rather than fever duration) and on 10 mg of prednisone chronically (2 points) would score 5 points for this section. The score for this section is recorded in box C on both sides of the PG-SGA form (Figures 2.1 and 2.2)

Scoring the Nutrition-related Physical Exam

The assessment of nutriture as determined by the physical exam is not based on a true point system. Each site examined (see figure 2.3, Table 4) is rated and then each aspect (adipose, muscle, and fluid status) is scored globally as follows:

    no deficit = 0
    mild deficit = 1 +
    moderate deficit = 2 ++
    severe deficit = 3 +++

Figure 2.2, Table 4 presents a worksheet to record data from the physical exam, as well as the global rating for fat, muscle, and fluid. The point score for the physical exam is determined by the overall subjective rating of total body deficit. Muscle deficit takes precedence over fat loss or fluid excess.

    no deficit = 0
    mild deficit = 1 point
    moderate deficit = 2 points
    severe deficit = 3 points

The numerical score for the physical exam is to be recorded in box D on Figure 2.1 and Figure 2.2, Table 4. Note: The point-score for physical exam should not exceed 3 points.

Triage for Medical Nutrition Therapy

Total numeric scores (of the first seven sections of the PG-SGA form, up to, and including the physical exam) are used to define specific nutrition intervention pathways such as education, symptom management, aggressive oral nutrition, and enteral/parenteral triage (see Chapter 3, *Medical Nutrition Therapy Protocols*).

<u>**A total additive total score of 0 to 1**</u> indicates that no intervention is required at this time and re-assessment on a regular and routine basis during treatment. Examples of patients with a total additive score of 0 to 1 are those:
- who have minimal weight loss within the past 1 month (<3% loss) or 6 months (<6%);
- who have been able to maintain or gain weight within the past 2 weeks and who are able to maintain this over time;
- who have no change or minimal change in their nutritional intake and have no nutrition impact symptoms or a single symptom scored as 1 point;
- who have minimal functional impairment.

<u>**A total additive score of 2 to 3**</u> is an indication for patient education by a dietetics professional or nurse, with pharmacologic triage by the nurse or physician as indicated by the apparent symptoms. Examples of patients falling within this category would include those with:
- 6% to 9.9% weight loss (alone, with no nutrition impact symptoms) within a 6-month period;
- 3% to 4.9% weight loss (alone, with no nutrition impact symptoms) within a 1-month period;
- mouth sores (alone);
- weight loss during past 2 weeks **and** 1) a 1-point nutrition impact symptom **or** 2) change in quantity of food intake **or** mild functional impairment;
- moderate functional impairment (symptomatic but spending less than 50% of time in bed or chair).

<u>**A total additive score of 4 to 8**</u> requires the intervention of the registered dietitian, working in conjunction with the nurse or physician as indicated by the symptom checklist for pharmacologic management. These would include any patient with at least one of the following:

- weight loss of ≥ 10% within the prior 6-month period
- weight loss of ≥ 5% within the prior 1-month period
- taking only liquids or nutritional supplements
- having checked off No Appetite, Vomiting, Diarrhea, or Pain
- chairbound or bedridden most or all of the day

A total additive score of 9 or greater indicates a critical need for symptom management and/or nutritional intervention. These are patients who require an interdisciplinary team meeting to address all aspects that are impacting the nutritional status as well as the potential need for non-oral nutritional options, including enteral or parenteral nutrition. This latter decision should be dictated by the presence or absence of a functioning gastrointestinal tract. It is important to note that symptom management is the first-line treatment of malnutrition. This may be accomplished using MNT and/or pharmacologic intervention. Aggressive symptom management is appropriate across the spectrum of cancer care.

How the Numeric Score Relates to Subjective Global Rating

Though the numeric score and subjective global rating are related, they are independent assessment and triage systems. In general, the higher total additive scores upon initial exam correlate with more severely malnourished cases. An example of a high numeric score that does not correlate with a severely or even moderately malnourished rating is the patient who is seen for the first time, and receives a numeric score of 14 and has a subjective global rating of *C* (severely malnourished). The same patient subsequently receives the appropriate medical nutrition therapy and pharmacologic intervention for nutrition impact symptoms. Upon follow-up, the patient is deemed to be anabolic (increase in nonfluid weight with improved intake), which is a subjective global rating of *A*, though still has a physical exam that suggests moderate to severe malnutrition.

Case Study

The following case study illustrates how the Scored PG-SGA is to be implemented. Figures 2.3 and 2.4 are examples of PG-SGA forms completed as they would be in the clinical setting. Follow the scenario of a 53-year-old male with squamous cell carcinoma of the larynx, who is being seen in the outpatient radiation therapy department. (It may be helpful to refer to the PG-SGA Scoring Guide section of this chapter.)

Our patient has completed the history portion (boxes 1–4) of the Scored PG-SGA in the waiting room (see Figure 2.3). The nurse clinician tabulates the score from the patient-generated information. Figure 2.4, Table 1 is a scoring guide for weight loss. Two points are scored for subacute weight loss (4.4%) over the past month and added to 1 point scored for acute weight loss over the past 2 weeks, for a total of 3 points.

In the Food Intake section (box 2), the patient has indicated that he is taking less than usual (1 point) and is taking little solid food (2 points). The score is the highest point value, not an additive score, and is therefore a 2. The score for Symptoms (box 3) is additive. The patient checked problems swallowing (2 points), pain (3 points), and dry mouth (1), for a total of 6 points. Activities and Function (box 4) was noted to be normal, which produces a zero score. The additive score of boxes 1–4 is 11, which is recorded is box A.

Figure 2.4, then Table 2 provide scoring for Disease and/or Condition. Note that only 1 point is generated in this section and is recorded in the corresponding box B in the lower-right-hand corner of Table 2 and on Figure 2.3. The medical record indicates that the patient is not taking any steroids and is afebrile, suggesting no metabolic stress, as noted on Figure 2.4, Table 3 Worksheet. A zero is recorded in box C in the table and on Figure 2.3.

Next, the nurse clinician performs a physical exam. The assessment of each of the sites examined is recorded on Figure 2.4, Table 4 Worksheet. The exam revealse that even though the under-eye fat pads were mildly depleted (1+), the global assessment (see Figure 2.4, Table 4 Worksheet) for fat stores is a zero because the fat stores in the triceps and anterior lower ribs were normal (0). The global, or overall, score for muscle stores is also a zero, as five out of seven sites examined reflected adequate (0) nutriture (see Figure 2.4, Table 4 Worksheet). Lastly, the global score for fluid status is a zero, as the ankles and sacrum were not edematous (0) and there was no ascites (0) (see Figure 2.4, Table 4 Worksheet). Overall, the patient has little sign of nutritional deficit, therefore, scoring zero points for the physical exam. A zero is recorded in box D in Figure 2.4, Table 4 Worksheet and on Figure 2.3.

The total numeric score of boxes A, B, C, and D for this case is 12 points. According to the Nutritional Triage recommendations given at the bottom of Figure 2.3, this indicates a critical need for improved symptom management and/or nutrient intervention opeionts (see Chapter 3, *Medical Nutrition Therapy Protocols;* Chapter 7, *Nutrition Concerns with the Radiation Therapy Patient;* Chapter 11, *Enteral Nutrition in Adult Medical/Surgical Oncology;* and Appendixes A and B). Despite having a large PG-SGA numerical score, Figure 2.4, Table 5 Worksheet shows the patient's global assessment is a B.

Summary

The Scored PG-SGA is an efficient and cost-effective tool to be used in nutrition assessment and triage of medical nutrition therapy (see Chapter 3) (11). Moreover, it is applicable in a variety of health care settings and is well-suited for use in multidisciplinary patient care. Proper training is essential prior to implementing the Scored PG-SGA, however. The video *Patient-Generated Subjective Global Assessment* provides viewers with step-by-step instruction in all the components of the PG-SGA, including physical examination and scoring (14). All of the necessary forms are included in the literature accompanying the video, allowing the viewer to follow along with the instruction.

Figure 2.1   Scored Patient-Generated Subjective Global Assessment (PG-SGA)

Scored Patient-Generated Subjective Global Assessment (PG-SGA)

Patient ID Information

History

1. Weight *(See Table 1 Worksheet)*

In summary of my current and recent weight:

I currently weigh about _____ pounds
I am about _____ feet _____ tall

One month ago I weighed about _____ pounds
Six months ago I weighed about _____ pounds

During the past two weeks my weight has:

☐ decreased $_{(1)}$ ☐ not changed $_{(0)}$ ☐ increased $_{(0)}$ ☐

2. Food Intake: As compared to my normal, I would rate my food intake during the past month as:
☐ unchanged (0)
☐ more than usual
☐ less than usual (1)
   I am now taki*ng:*
     ☐ *normal food* but less than normal (1)
     ☐ little solid food (2)
     ☐ only liquids (3)
     ☐ only nutritonal supplements (3)
     ☐ very little of anything $_{(4)}$
     ☐ only tube feedings or only nutrition by vein ☐

3. Symptoms: I have had the following problems that have kept me from eating enough during the past two weeks (check all that apply):
☐ no problems eating $_{(0)}$
☐ no appetite, just did not feel like eating $_{(3)}$

☐ nausea $_{(1)}$ ☐ vomiting $_{(3)}$
☐ constipation $_{(1)}$ ☐ diarrhea $_{(3)}$
☐ mouth sores $_{(2)}$ ☐ dry mouth $_{(1)}$
☐ things taste funny or have no taste $_{(1)}$ ☐ smells bother me $_{(1)}$
☐ problems swallowing $_{(2)}$ ☐ feel full quickly $_{(1)}$
☐ pain; where? $_{(3)}$ _____
☐ other** $_{(1)}$ _____
   ** Examples: depression, money, or dental problems ☐

4. Activities and Function: Over the past month, I would generally rate my activity as:
☐ normal with no limitations $_{(0)}$
☐ not my normal self, but able to be up and about with fairly normal activities $_{(1)}$
☐ not feeling up to most things, but in bed less than half the day $_{(2)}$
☐ able to do little activity and spend most of the day in bed or chair $_{(3)}$

Additive Score of the Boxes 1-4 ☐ **A**

The remainder of this form will be complete by your doctor, nurse, or therapist. Thank you.

5. Disease and its relation to nutritional requirements *(See Table 2)*

All relevant diagnoses (specify) _____

Primary disease stage (circle if known or appropriate)   I   II   III   IV   Other _____

Age _____

Numerical score from Table 2 ☐ **B**

6. Metabolic Demand *(See Table 3 Worksheet)*
☐ no stress   ☐ low stress   ☐ moderate stress   ☐ high stress

Numerical score from Table 3 ☐ **C**

7. Physical *(See Table 4 Worksheet)*

Numerical score from Table 4 ☐ **D**

Global Assessment *(See Table 5 Worksheet)*
☐ Well-nourished or anabolic (SGA-A)
☐ Moderate or suspected malnutrition (SGA-B)
☐ Severely malnourished (SGA-C)

Total numerical score of boxes A+B+C+D ☐
(See triage recommendations below)

Clinician Signature _____ RD RN PA MD DO Other ___   Date _____

Nutritional Triage Recommendations: Additive score is used to define specific nutritional interventions including patient & family education, symptom management including pharmacologic intervention, and appropriate nutrient intervention (food, nutritional supplements, enteral, or parenteral triage). First line nutrition intervention includes optimal symptom management.

0-1   No intervention required at this time. Re-assessment on routine and regular basis during treatment.
2-3   Patient & family education by dietitian, nurse, or other clinician with pharmacologic intervention as indicated by symptom survey (Box 3) and laboratory values as appropriate.
4-8   Requires intervention by dietitian, in conjunction with nurse or physician, as indicated by symptoms survey (Box 3).
≥ 9   Indicates a critical need for improved symptom management and/or nutrient intervention options.

Figure 2.2   Tables and Worksheets for PG-SGA Scoring

Tables & Worksheets for PG-SGA Scoring

The PG-SGA numerical score is derived by totaling the scores from boxes A-D of the PG-SGA on the reverse side. Boxes 1-4 are designed to be completed by the patient. The points assigned to items in boxes 1-4 are noted parenthetically after each item. The following worksheets are offered as aids for calcuating scores of sections that are not so marked.

Table 1 - Scoring Weight (wt) Loss

Determined by adding points for subacute and acute wt change. **Subacute:** If information is available about weight loss during past 1 month, add the point score to the points for acute wt change. Only include the wt loss over 6 months if the wt from 1 month is unavailable. **Acute:** refers to wt change during past two weeks. Add 1 point to subacute score if patient lost wt; add no points if patient gained or maintained wt during the past two weeks.

Wt loss in 1 month	Points	Wt loss in 6 months
10% or greater	4	20% or greater
5-9.9%	3	10 -19.9%
3-4.9%	2	6 - 9.9%
2-2.9%	1	2 - 5.9%
0-1.9%	0	0 - 1.9%

Points for Box 1 = Subacute + Acute = ☐

Table 2 - Scoring criteria for disease &/or condition

Score is derived by adding 1 point for each of the conditions listed below that pertain to the patient.

Category	Points
Cancer	1
AIDS	1
Pulmonary or cardiac cachexia	1
Presence of decubitus, open wound, or fistula	1
Presence of trauma	1
Age greater than 65 years	1

Points for Box 2 = ☐ B

Table 3 Worksheet. Scoring Metabolic Stress

Score for metabolic stress is determined by a number of variables known to increase protein & calorie needs. The score is additive so that a patient who has a fever of > 102 degrees (3 points) and is on 10 mg of prednisone chronically (2 points) would have an additive score for this section of 5 points.

Stress	none (0)	low (1)	moderate (2)	high (3)
Fever	no fever	>99 and <101	≥101 and <102	≥102
Fever duration	no fever	<72 hrs	72 hrs	> 72 hrs
Steroids	no steroids	low dose (<10mg prednisone equivalents/day)	moderate dose (≥10 and <30mg prednisone equivalents/day)	high dose steroids (≥30mg prednisone equivalents/day)

Points for Table 3 = ☐ C

Table 4 Worksheet - Physical Examination

Physical exam includes a subjective evaluation of 3 aspects of body composition: fat, muscle, & fluid status. Since this is subjective, each aspect of the exam is rated for degree of deficit. Definition of categories: 0 = no deficit, 1+ = mild deficit, 2+ = moderate deficit, 3+ = severe deficit. Degree of muscle deficit takes precedence over fat deficit. Rating of deficit in these categories are *not* additive but a used to clinically assess the degree of deficit (or presence of excess fluid).

Fat Stores:

orbital fat pads	0	1+	2+	3+
triceps skin fold	0	1+	2+	3+
fat overlying lower ribs	0	1+	2+	3+
Global fat deficit rating	**0**	**1+**	**2+**	**3+**

Fluid Status:

ankle edema	0	1+	2+	3+
sacral edema	0	1+	2+	3+
ascites	0	1+	2+	3+
Global fluid status rating	**0**	**1+**	**2+**	**3+**

Muscle Status:

temples (temporalis muscle)	0	1+	2+	3+
clavicles (pectoralis & deltoids)	0	1+	2+	3+
shoulders (deltoids)	0	1+	2+	3+
interosseous muscles	0	1+	2+	3+
scapula (latissimus dorsi, trapezius, deltoids)	0	1+	2+	3+
thigh (quadriceps)	0	1+	2+	3+
calf (gastrocnemius)	0	1+	2+	3+
Global muscle status rating	**0**	**1+**	**2+**	**3+**

Point score for the physical exam is determined by the overall subjective rating of total body deficit; again muscle deficit takes precedence over fat loss or fluid excess.

No deficit	score = 0 points
Mild deficit	score = 1 point
Moderate deficit	score = 2 points
Severe deficit	score = 3 points

Points for Worksheet 4 = ☐ D

Table 5 Worksheet PG-SGA Global Assessment Categories

Category	Stage A — Well-nourished	Stage B — Moderately malnourished or suspected malnutrition	Stage C — Severely malnourished
Weight	No wt loss **or** Recent non-fluid wt gain	~5% wt loss within 1 month (or 10% in 6 months) No wt stabilization or wt gain (i.e., continued wt loss)	a. > 5% loss in 1 month (or >10% loss in 6 months) b. No wt stabilization or wt gain (i.e., continued wt loss)
Nutrient Intake	No deficit **or** Significant recent improvement	Definite decrease in intake	Severe deficit in intake
Nutrition Impact Symptoms	None **or** Significant recent improvement allowing adequate intake	Presence of nutrition impact symptoms (Box 3 of PG-SGA)	Presence of nutrition impact symptoms (Box 3 of PG-SGA)
Functioning	No deficit **or** Significant recent improvement	Moderate functional deficit **or** Recent deterioration	Severe functional deficit **or** recent significant deterioration
Physical Exam	No deficit **or** Chronic deficit but with recent clinical improvement	Evidence of mild to moderate loss of SQ fat &/or muscle mass &/or muscle tone on palpation	Obvious signs of malnutrition (e.g., severe loss of SQ tissues, possible edema)

Global PG-SGA rating (A, B, or C) = ☐

Figure 2.3   Scored Patient-Generated Subjective Global Assessment (PG-SGA) (completed example)

Scored Patient-Generated Subjective Global Assessment (PG-SGA)

Patient ID Information

History

1. Weight *(See Table 1 Worksheet)*

In summary of my current and recent weight:

I currently weigh about __175__ pounds
I am about __6__ feet __1__ tall

One month ago I weighed about __183__ pounds
Six months ago I weighed about __?__ pounds

During the past two weeks my weight has:

☒ decreased $_{(1)}$ ☐ not changed $_{(0)}$ ☐ increased $_{(0)}$

3

2. Food Intake: As compared to my normal, I would rate my food intake during the past month as:
☐ unchanged (0)
☐ more than usual
☒ less than usual (1)
I am now tak*ing:*
  ☐ *normal food* but less than normal (1)
  ☒ little solid food (2)
  ☐ only liquids (3)
  ☐ only nutritonal supplements (3)
  ☐ very little of anything $_{(4)}$
  ☐ only tube feedings or only nutrition by vein

2

3. Symptoms: I have had the following problems that have kept me from eating enough during the past two weeks (check all that apply):
☐ no problems eating $_{(0)}$
☐ no appetite, just did not feel like eating $_{(3)}$

☐ nausea $_{(1)}$ ☐ vomiting $_{(3)}$
☐ constipation $_{(1)}$ ☐ diarrhea $_{(3)}$
☐ mouth sores $_{(2)}$ ☒ dry mouth $_{(1)}$
☐ things taste funny or have no taste $_{(1)}$ ☐ smells bother me $_{(1)}$
☒ problems swallowing $_{(2)}$ ☐ feel full quickly $_{(1)}$
☒ pain; where? $_{(3)}$ *throat*
☐ other** $_{(1)}$ _____
** Examples: depression, money, or dental problems

6

4. Activities and Function: Over the past month, I would generally rate my activity as:
☒ normal with no limitations $_{(0)}$
☐ not my normal self, but able to be up and about with fairly normal activities $_{(1)}$
☐ not feeling up to most things, but in bed less than half the day $_{(2)}$
☐ able to do little activity and spend most of the day in bed or chair $_{(3)}$

0

Additive Score of the Boxes 1-4 **11** **A**

The remainder of this form will be complete by your doctor, nurse, or therapist. Thank you.

5. Disease and its relation to nutritional requirements *(See Table 2)*
All relevant diagnoses (specify) _squamous cell carcinoma of the larynx_____

Primary disease stage (circle if known or appropriate)   I   II   III   IV   Other _____

Age **53**

Numerical score from Table 2 **1** **B**

6. Metabolic Demand *(See Table 3 Worksheet)*
☒ no stress   ☐ low stress   ☐ moderate stress   ☐ high stress

Numerical score from Table 3 **0** **C**

7. Physical *(See Table 4 Worksheet)*

Numerical score from Table 4 **0** **D**

Global Assessment *(See Table 5 Worksheet)*
☐ Well-nourished or anabolic (SGA-A)
☒ Moderate or suspected malnutrition (SGA-B)
☐ Severely malnourished (SGA-C)

Total numerical score of boxes A+B+C+D **12**
(See triage recommendations below)

Clinician Signature _____ RD RN PA MD DO Other ___   Date _____

Nutritional Triage Recommendations: Additive score is used to define specific nutritional interventions including patient & family education, symptom management including pharmacologic intervention, and appropriate nutrient intervention (food, nutritional supplements, enteral, or parenteral triage). First line nutrition intervention includes optimal symptom management.

0-1   No intervention required at this time. Re-assessment on routine and regular basis during treatment.
2-3   Patient & family education by dietitian, nurse, or other clinician with pharmacologic intervention as indicated by symptom survey (Box 3) and laboratory values as appropriate.
4-8   Requires intervention by dietitian, in conjunction with nurse or physician, as indicated by symptoms survey (Box 3).
≥9   Indicates a critical need for improved symptom management and/or nutrient intervention options.

Figure 2.4   Tables and Worksheets for PG-SGA Scoring (completed example)

Tables & Worksheets for PG-SGA Scoring

The PG-SGA numerical score is derived by totaling the scores from boxes A-D of the PG-SGA on the reverse side. Boxes 1-4 are designed to be completed by the patient. The points assigned to items in boxes 1-4 are noted parenthetically after each item. The following worksheets are offered as aids for calcuating scores of sections that are not so marked.

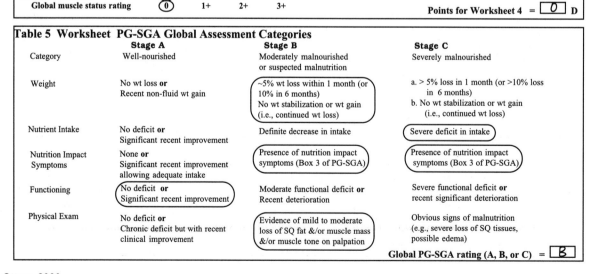

Table 1 - Scoring Weight (wt) Loss

Determined by adding points for subacute and acute wt change. **Subacute**: If information is available about weight loss during past 1 month, add the point score to the points for acute wt change. Only include the wt loss over 6 months if the wt from 1 month is unavailable. **Acute**: refers to wt change during past two weeks. Add 1 point to subacute score if patient lost wt; add no points if patient gained or maintained wt during the past two weeks.

Wt loss in 1 month	Points	Wt loss in 6 months
10% or greater	4	20% or greater
5-9.9%	3	10 -19.9%
(3-4.9%)	(2)	6 - 9.9%
2-2.9%	1	2 - 5.9%
0-1.9%	0	0 - 1.9%

Points for Box 1 = Subacute + Acute = `3`

Table 2 - Scoring criteria for disease &/or condition

Score is derived by adding 1 point for each of the conditions listed below that pertain to the patient.

Category	Points
Cancer	(1)
AIDS	1
Pulmonary or cardiac cachexia	1
Presence of decubitus, open wound, or fistula	1
Presence of trauma	1
Age greater than 65 years	1

Points for Table 2 = `1` B

Table 3 Worksheet. Scoring Metabolic Stress

Score for metabolic stress is determined by a number of variables known to increase protein & calorie needs. The score is additive so that a patient who has a fever of > 102 degrees (3 points) and is on 10 mg of prednisone chronically (2 points) would have an additive score for this section of 5 points.

Stress	none (0)	low (1)	moderate (2)	high (3)
Fever	no fever	>99 and <101	≥101 and <102	≥102
Fever duration	no fever	<72 hrs	72 hrs	> 72 hrs
Steroids	no steroids	low dose (<10mg prednisone equivalents/day)	moderate dose (≥10 and <30mg prednisone equivalents/day)	high dose steroids (≥30mg prednisone equivalents/day)

Points for Table 3 = `0` C

Table 4 Worksheet - Physical Examination

Physical exam includes a subjective evaluation of 3 aspects of body composition: fat, muscle, & fluid status. Since this is subjective, each aspect of the exam is rated for degree of deficit. Definition of categories: 0 = no deficit, 1+ = mild deficit, 2+ = moderate deficit, 3+ = severe deficit. Degree of muscle deficit takes precedence over fat deficit. Rating of deficit in these categories are *not* additive but a used to clinically assess the degree of deficit (or presence of excess fluid).

Fat Stores:

orbital fat pads	0	(1+)	2+	3+
triceps skin fold	(0)	1+	2+	3+
fat overlying lower ribs	(0)	1+	2+	3+
Global fat deficit rating	(0)	1+	2+	3+

Muscle Status:

temples (temporalis muscle)	0	(1+)	2+	3+
clavicles (pectoralis & deltoids)	0	(1+)	2+	3+
shoulders (deltoids)	(0)	1+	2+	3+
interosseous muscles	(0)	1+	2+	3+
scapula (latissimus dorsi, trapezius, deltoids)	(0)	1+	2+	3+
thigh (quadriceps)	(0)	1+	2+	3+
calf (gastrocnemius)	(0)	1+	2+	3+
Global muscle status rating	(0)	1+	2+	3+

Fluid Status:

ankle edema	(0)	1+	2+	3+
sacral edema	(0)	1+	2+	3+
ascites	(0)	1+	2+	3+
Global fluid status rating	(0)	1+	2+	3+

Point score for the physical exam is determined by the overall subjective rating of total body deficit; again muscle deficit takes precedence over fat loss or fluid excess.

No deficit	score = 0 points
Mild deficit	score = 1 point
Moderate deficit	score = 2 points
Severe deficit	score = 3 points

Points for Worksheet 4 = `0` D

Table 5 Worksheet PG-SGA Global Assessment Categories

Category	Stage A Well-nourished	Stage B Moderately malnourished or suspected malnutrition	Stage C Severely malnourished
Weight	No wt loss **or** Recent non-fluid wt gain	~5% wt loss within 1 month (or 10% in 6 months) No wt stabilization or wt gain (i.e., continued wt loss)	a. > 5% loss in 1 month (or >10% loss in 6 months) b. No wt stabilization or wt gain (i.e., continued wt loss)
Nutrient Intake	No deficit **or** Significant recent improvement	Definite decrease in intake	Severe deficit in intake
Nutrition Impact Symptoms	None **or** Significant recent improvement allowing adequate intake	Presence of nutrition impact symptoms (Box 3 of PG-SGA)	Presence of nutrition impact symptoms (Box 3 of PG-SGA)
Functioning	No deficit **or** Significant recent improvement	Moderate functional deficit **or** Recent deterioration	Severe functional deficit **or** recent significant deterioration
Physical Exam	No deficit **or** Chronic deficit but with recent clinical improvement	Evidence of mild to moderate loss of SQ fat &/or muscle mass &/or muscle tone on palpation	Obvious signs of malnutrition (e.g., severe loss of SQ tissues, possible edema)

Global PG-SGA rating (A, B, or C) = `B`

References

1. Joint Commission on Accreditation of Healthcare Organizations Comprehensive Accreditation Manual for Hospitals: The Official Handbook. Oakbrook Terrace, Ill: JCAHO; 1999.

2. 1999-2000 Comprehensive Accreditation Manual for Homecare (CAMHC). Oakbrook Terrace, Ill: JCAHO; 1999.

3. Ottery, FD, Kasenic, S, DeBolt, S, Rodgers, K. Volunteer network accrues >1900 patients in 6 months to validate standardized nutritional triage. *Proceedings of ASCO*. 1998, 17:abstract 282.

4. Detsky AS, Baker JP, Mendelson RA, Wolman SL, Wesson DE, Jeejeebhoy KN. Evaluating the accuracy of nutritional assessment techniques applied to hospitalized patients: methodology and comparisons. *JPEN*. 1984; 8(2):153-159.

5. Detsky AS, McLaughlin JR, Baker JP, Johnston N, Whittaker S,. Mendelson RA, Jeejeebhoy KN. What is subjective global assessment of nutritional status? *JPEN*. 1987; 11(1):8-13.

6. Hirsch S, de Obadia N, Petermann M, Rojo P, Barrientos C, Iturriaga H, Bunout D. Subjective global assessment of nutritional status: Further validation. *Nutrition*. 1991:7;35-37.

7. Baker JP, Detsky AS, Wesson DE, Wolman SL, Stewart S, Whitewell JB, Jeejeebhoy KN. A comparison of clinical judgement and objective measurements. *NEJM*. 1982; 306:969.

8. Detsky AS, Baker JP, O'Rourke K, Johnston N, Whitwell J, Mendelson RA, Jeejeebhoy KN. Predicting nutrition-associated complications for patients undergoing gastrointestinal surgery. *JPEN*. 1987;11:444-446.

9. Ottery FD. Rethinking nutritional support of the cancer patient: the new field of nutritional oncology. *Sem Oncol*. 1994;21:770-778.

10. McMahon, K, Decker, G, Ottery, FD. Integrating proactive nutritional assessment in clinical practices to prevent complications and cost. *Sem Oncol*. 1998; 25(No 2, Suppl 6):20-27.

11. Smith KG (ed). *Medical Nutrition Therapy Across the Continuum of Care*. 2nd ed. Chicago, Ill: The American Dietetic Association; 1998.

12. Ottery FD. Oncology patient-generated SGA of nutritional status. *Nutr Onc*. 1994;1(2):9.

13. Blackburn GL, Bistrian BR, Maini BS. Nutritional and metabolic assessment of the hospitalized patient. *JPEN* 1977;1:11-22.

14. McCallum PD, Polisena CG, Kulakowski K. Patient-Generated Subjective Global Assessment [videotape]. Chicago, Ill: The American Dietetic Association; 2000.

Suggested Reading

Perioperative total parenteral nutrition in surgical patients. The Veterans Affairs Total Parental Nutrition Cooperative Study Group. *NEJM*. 1991; 325(8):525-532.

Enia G, Sicuso C, Alati G, Zoccali C. Subjective global assessment of nutrition in dialysis patients. *Nephrol Dial Transplant*. 1993; 8(10):1094-1098.

Hasse J, Gorman MA, Liepa G. Subjective global assessment: alternative nutrition-assessment technique for liver-transplant candidates. *Nutrition*. 1993; 9:339.

Newton JM, Halsted CH. Clinical and Functional Assessment of Adults. In: Shils ME, Olsen JA, Shike M, and Ross AC, eds. Modern nutrition. In: *Health and Disease*. 9th ed. Baltimore, Md: Williams and Wilkins; 1999:895-902.

McLeod RS, Taylor BR, O'Connor BL, Greenberg GR, Jeejeebhoy KN, Royall D, Langer B. Quality of life, nutritional status, and gastrointestinal hormone profile following Whipple procedure. *Am J Surg*. 1995; 169:179-185.

Ottery FD. Cancer cachexia: prevention, early diagnosis, and management. *Cancer Practice*. 1994; 2(2):123-131.

Ottery FD. Nutritional screening and assessment in the homecare setting. *Infusion*. 1996;2:36-45.

Ottery FD. Nutritional oncology: an integrated approach to the cancer patient. In: Shikora S and Blackburn GL, eds. *Nutrition Support: Theory and Therapeutics*. New York: Chapman and Hall; 1997.

3

Medical Nutrition Therapy Protocols

Sandra Luthringer, RD   **Karen Kulakowski, MA, RD, CNSD**

Over the past decade, emphasis has been placed on evaluating the effectiveness of nutrition services to curb rising health care costs. Practice guidelines, which dietetics professionals developed, have been the standard of care in most institutions. While practice guidelines provide standardized recommendations for care, they do not always specify timelines or expected outcomes. Thus, the need for measurable outcome-based research arose.

Medical Nutrition Therapy (MNT) is defined as a planned series of activities which, when provided to a given population, will result in a change in behavior, risk factor, status of health or need for health care resources. The goal of MNT is a measurable outcome.

Development of Medical Nutrition Therapy Protocols

The Medical Nutrition Therapy Patient Protocols were a collaborative effort of various committees within The American Dietetic Association. These include several dietetic practice groups, the Quality Management Committee, the Reimbursement Committee, and the Headquarters teams. Many experienced clinicians affiliated with Morrison Health Care, Cambridge Health Alliance, and the United States Department of Defense made significant contributions. Additionally, the editors of this book and the authors of this chapter were involved in the development of the protocols. These organizations and individuals have defined protocols as detailed guidelines for care specific to disease or condition and to type of patient. These protocols define MNT in concrete terms, increase effectiveness of care by promoting consistency, and provide clearer measurements of quality and effectiveness of care. The protocols are also compatible with current trends in health care financing. (1)

The changes that are presently occurring in the national health care system present unique challenges and opportunities for dietetic professionals. Integrated health care systems or networks are emerging as a solution to the challenge of maintaining quality of care while containing costs. Health insurance plans and programs, health maintenance organizations (HMOs), and preferred provider organizations (PPOs) manage the allocation of health care benefits. Nutrition services may or may not be covered as part of basic medical care, but it is clear that unless a substantial cost savings to the insurer is shown, dietetic professionals will be passed over as important providers and an integral part of the medical care team. (2)

When evaluating outcomes of nutrition care, it is important to have a clear understanding of both the objectives that determine the selection of outcome criteria and who is defining the objectives. This will assure that the objectives clearly reflect the population studied. For example, many studies of cancer treatments have focused solely on survival rates, regardless of the quality of life experienced by patients. While survival rates are an important outcome of treatment, quality of life may be a more appropriate outcome of nutrition intervention during cancer treatment. With this in mind, the findings of outcome research will provide insight, guide clinical practice, and determine benchmarks for measuring quality of care.

The MNT protocols for oncology were developed through a consultative process by experts and practitioners. They incorporate current professional knowledge and available research and clearly define the level, content, and frequency of nutritional care. Two MNT protocols are included in this chapter: the Medical Oncology Protocols and Radiation Oncology Protocols.

The protocols are meant to serve as a general framework for counseling patients with particular health problems, and it may not always be appropriate to use them to manage patients. Individual circumstances vary and can require actions that differ from these protocols. The independent skill and judgment of the dietetics professional must always dictate treatment decisions. The protocols do not establish or specify particular standards of care, whether legal, medical, or other. (3)

The oncology protocols are not yet field-tested. However, they have been reviewed for content and accuracy by physicians, certified registered nurse practitioners, and several registered dietitians, all practicing in the area of oncology. A third edition of *Medical Nutrition Therapy Across the Continuum of Care* is expected in 2001.

Organization of Protocols (1)

Each protocol is organized into five sections:
- Summary Page
- Flowchart
- Session Process
- Nutrition Progress Notes
- Bibliography

Summary Page (Figures 3.1a and 3.1b)

This page summarizes the entire process. It includes the number of interventions, expected length of time for each intervention, and costs or charges when required by payers. The second portion summarizes the expected outcomes of the MNT. Outcomes are defined as the result of the performance, or nonperformance, of the patient to a specific function or process. Outcome assessment factors include the following:

- **Clinical Assessment** measures anatomic and physiologic elements, such as biochemical parameters, anthropometric parameters, and clinical signs and symptoms.
- **Functional Assessment** measures physical capability, such as activities of daily living, social functioning, and mental/emotional health for diagnosis or conditions.
- **Behavioral Assessment** measures changes in the patient's behavior related to food selections, preparation, and activity that will ultimately result in changes in clinical or functional outcomes.

Included on this summary page are the expected outcomes, which indicate the anticipated change and the ideal or goal value, which lists what is to be considered appropriate for control or improvement.

Flowchart (Figures 3.2a and 3.2b)

The flowchart is a one-page visual overview of the process, including specific data to be obtained prior to the initial session, data to be assessed, self-management training expectations by session, and communications to the appropriate health care provider.

Session Process (Figures 3.3a and 3.3b)

This section provides details of the oncology protocols by session for the dietetic professional. Specific factors to be covered in this session are divided into three sections:

- **Assessment** includes, but is not limited to, an accurate and current nutrition history, a lifestyle assessment, and the patient's knowledge base and willingness to learn. Refer to Chapter 2, *Patient-Generated Subjective Global Assessment,* for detailed direction on performing a physical assessment.
- **Intervention** begins with the identification of treatment goals and the development of individualized nutrition care plans.
- **Communication** is an important aspect of the session and involves the client, caregiver, primary care provider, oncologist and/or other members of the health care team as needed.

Nutrition Progress Notes (Figures 3.4a and 3.4b)

The notes are specific to oncology and are designed to document the intervention and outcomes of MNT outlined in the session process. This section contains a simple format for documenting expected outcome, intervention provided to meet the goals, and whether each goal was reached or not. Communication skills are an important factor in the success of these protocols. Information regarding expected outcomes and goals must be shared with the patient and the referring provider, and documented in the medical record.

Bibliography (Figure 3.5)

The comprehensive bibliography is based on nationally recognized peer-reviewed journals supporting the content of these protocols.

Summary

The MNT Protocols reflect the new practice of dietetics. As the science of nutrition changes, dietetics practice must conform to reflect new knowledge. By utilizing standardized protocols, dietetics professionals will have the opportunity to share the benefits of MNT with administrators, physicians, and third-party payers. These benefits include improved outcomes, shorter length of stay, and cost savings to benefit not only the patient, but the institution, the clinician, and third-party payers.

References

1. Gillbreath J, Inman-Felton AE, Johnson EQ, Robinson G, Smith KG (eds). *Medical Nutrition Therapy Across the Continuum of Care—Client Protocols.* 2nd ed. Chicago, Ill: The American Dietetic Association; 1998.
2. Stollman L (ed). *Nutrition Entrepreneur's Guide to Reimbursement Success* 2nd ed. Chicago, Ill: The American Dietetic Association; 1999.

Note: The Medical Nutrition Therapy Protocol forms contained in this book may be reproduced for professional use.

Figure 3.1a Cancer (Medical) Summary Page

CANCER (MEDICAL)
Medical Nutrition Therapy Protocol

Setting: Medical Oncology Ambulatory Care or adapted for other settings (Adult 18+ years old)
Note: Same principles can be used for surgical oncology clients.
Number of sessions: varies with PG-SGA.*

No. of interventions	Length of contact	Time between interventions	Cost/charge
1	60 minutes	As identified from PG-SGA*	
2	30 minutes	As identified from PG-SGA*	
3	15-30 minutes	As identified from PG-SGA*	

*Patient-Generated Subjective Global Assessment.

Expected Outcomes of Medical Nutrition Therapy

Outcome assessment factors	Baseline	Evaluation of Intervention Interventions			Expected outcome	Ideal/goal value
		1	2	3		
Clinical						
• Biochemical parameters Albumin Prealbumin CBC Absolute neutrophil count (ANC) SMA12 (includes electrolytes, Ca, Mg, P, BUN, creatinine, LFT, glucose)	✔ ✔ ✔ ✔ ✔ ✔				Labs repeated based on client's condition	Albumin 3.5-5.0 g/dL Prealbumin 19-43 mg/gL HgB >12 g/dL (F) >14 g/dL (M) Hct >38 vol% (F) >44 vol% (M) ANC >500
• Anthropometrics Weight, height, BMI, UBW • Clinical signs and symptoms (eg, nausea, bowel changes, esophagitis)	✔ ✔	✔ ✔	✔ ✔		Weight maintenance to <1% of actual weight/week Prevent dehydration Minimize severity of side effects of ≤ grade 2 on Chemotherapy Toxicity Criteria	SMA12 within normal limits Maintain wt to ≥85% UBW Toxicity ≤ grade 2 on Chemotherapy Toxicity Criteria
Functional Perform ADLs	✔	✔	✔		Maintain PO adequate to perform ADLs per Chemotherapy Toxicity Criteria	Intake adequate to maintain ADLs
Behavioral* • Oral intake adequate to maintain nutritional status • Knowledge of high-calorie/protein foods/supplements • Knowledge of foods to include/avoid based on side effects of treatment • Knowledge of potential food/drug interactions • Knowledge of complementary nutritional therapies (eg, herb preparations, megadose vitamin treatment) • Knowledge of nutrition supplements and alternative feeding routes • Knowledge of healthy eating habits and diet, nutrition, and cancer prevention recommendations	✔ ✔ ✔	✔ ✔ ✔ ✔ ✔ ✔ ✔	✔ ✔ ✔ ✔ ✔ ✔ ✔		• Verbalizes importance of appropriate nutrition • Consumes high-calorie/protein foods • Consumes foods that lessen side effects of treatment • Avoids foods that may cause side effects with treatment • Uses appropriate/safe complementary nutrition therapies • Uses appropriate supplements as needed • Uses acceptable alternative feeding routes, such as enteral feedings, if oral intake not adequate • Uses individualized eating plan, making healthy food choices and using diet, nutrition, and cancer prevention recommendations	**MNT Goals** • Maintain adequate intake of calories and protein • Select foods to limit side effects of treatment • Maintain stable weight • After treatments, adopt healthy eating plans

*Session in which behavioral topics are covered may vary according to client's/caregiver's readiness, skills, resources, and need for lifestyle changes.

Medical Nutrition Therapy Across the Continuum of Care

Figure 3.1b Cancer (Radiation Oncology) Summary Page

CANCER (RADIATION ONCOLOGY)
Medical Nutrition Therapy Protocol

Setting: Ambulatory Care or adapted for other health care settings (Adult 18+ years old)
Number of sessions: 3

No. of interventions	Length of contact	Time between interventions	Cost/charge
1	30-60 minutes	As identified from PG-SGA*	
2a (head/neck/pelvic irradiation clients)	15-30 minutes	1 week	
2b (all clients other than 2a)	15-30 minutes	2 weeks	
3	15-30 minutes	Weekly as needed	

*Patient-Generated Subjective Global Assessment.

Expected Outcomes of Medical Nutrition Therapy

Outcome assessment factors	Base-line	Evaluation of Intervention 1	2	3	Expected outcome	Ideal/goal value
Clinical • Biochemical parameters Laboratory results as available	✔	✔		✔		
• Anthropometrics Weight, height, BMI, UBW	✔	✔		✔	Minimize weight loss to <1% of actual weight/week	Maintain weight to ≥85% usual body weight
Clinical signs and symptoms (eg, nausea, bowel changes)	✔	✔		✔	Minimize severity of side effects to ≤ grade 2 on Chemotherapy Toxicity Criteria	Toxicity to ≤ grade 2 on Chemotherapy Toxicity Criteria
Functional Perform ADLs	✔	✔		✔	Maintain PO adequate to perform ADLs per Chemotherapy Toxicity Criteria	Intake adequate to maintain ADLs
Behavioral* • Oral intake adequate to maintain weight	✔	✔		✔	• Verbalizes importance of adequate nutrition • Consumes adequate calories to meet expected weight and maintain goal • Maintains hydration status as measured by blood pressure within normal limits, good skin turgor, no signs of dehydration or dizziness	**MNT Goals** • Maintain adequate intake of calories and protein • Select foods to avoid side effects of treatment • After treatment, adopt individualized healthy eating plan
• Knowledge of high-calorie, high-protein supplements		✔		✔	• Consumes high-calorie, high-protein supplements, as needed	
• Knowledge of foods to avoid/include to ↓ side effects of treatment		✔		✔	• Consumes/avoids foods that lessen side effects of treatment	
• Knowledge of complementary nutrition therapies (eg, herb preparations, diets, vitamin supplements)		✔		✔	• Uses acceptable/safe complementary nutrition therapies	
• Knowledge of alternative mode of feeding (tube feeding), if indicated	✔	✔		✔	• Accepts/utilizes tube feeding to meet calorie/protein needs	
• Knowledge of healthy eating habits and diet, nutrition and cancer prevention recommendations				✔	• Uses individualized eating plan to make healthy food choices and follow diet, nutrition, and cancer prevention recommendations	

*Session in which behavioral topics are covered may vary according to client's/caregiver's readiness, skills, resources, and need for lifestyle changes.

Figure 3.2a Cancer (Medical) Flowchart Page

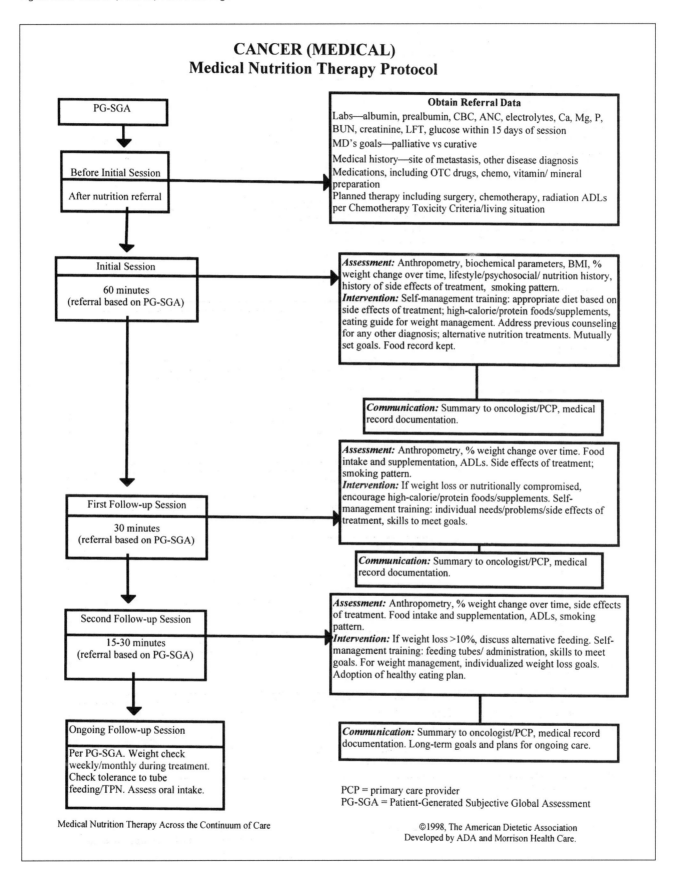

CANCER (MEDICAL)
Medical Nutrition Therapy Protocol

PG-SGA

Before Initial Session

After nutrition referral

Obtain Referral Data
Labs—albumin, prealbumin, CBC, ANC, electrolytes, Ca, Mg, P, BUN, creatinine, LFT, glucose within 15 days of session
MD's goals—palliative vs curative
Medical history—site of metastasis, other disease diagnosis
Medications, including OTC drugs, chemo, vitamin/ mineral preparation
Planned therapy including surgery, chemotherapy, radiation ADLs per Chemotherapy Toxicity Criteria/living situation

Initial Session

60 minutes
(referral based on PG-SGA)

Assessment: Anthropometry, biochemical parameters, BMI, % weight change over time, lifestyle/psychosocial/ nutrition history, history of side effects of treatment, smoking pattern.
Intervention: Self-management training: appropriate diet based on side effects of treatment; high-calorie/protein foods/supplements, eating guide for weight management. Address previous counseling for any other diagnosis; alternative nutrition treatments. Mutually set goals. Food record kept.

Communication: Summary to oncologist/PCP, medical record documentation.

First Follow-up Session

30 minutes
(referral based on PG-SGA)

Assessment: Anthropometry, % weight change over time. Food intake and supplementation, ADLs. Side effects of treatment; smoking pattern.
Intervention: If weight loss or nutritionally compromised, encourage high-calorie/protein foods/supplements. Self-management training: individual needs/problems/side effects of treatment, skills to meet goals.

Communication: Summary to oncologist/PCP, medical record documentation.

Second Follow-up Session

15-30 minutes
(referral based on PG-SGA)

Assessment: Anthropometry, % weight change over time, side effects of treatment. Food intake and supplementation, ADLs, smoking pattern.
Intervention: If weight loss >10%, discuss alternative feeding. Self-management training: feeding tubes/ administration, skills to meet goals. For weight management, individualized weight loss goals. Adoption of healthy eating plan.

Communication: Summary to oncologist/PCP, medical record documentation. Long-term goals and plans for ongoing care.

Ongoing Follow-up Session

Per PG-SGA. Weight check weekly/monthly during treatment. Check tolerance to tube feeding/TPN. Assess oral intake.

PCP = primary care provider
PG-SGA = Patient-Generated Subjective Global Assessment

Medical Nutrition Therapy Across the Continuum of Care

©1998, The American Dietetic Association
Developed by ADA and Morrison Health Care.

Figure 3.2b Cancer (Radiation Oncology) Flowchart Page

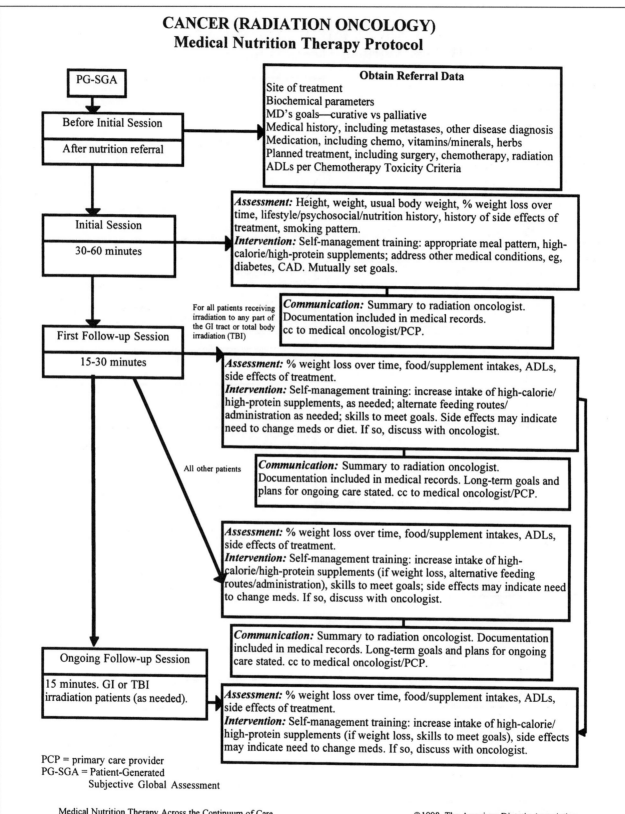

CANCER (RADIATION ONCOLOGY)
Medical Nutrition Therapy Protocol

PG-SGA

Before Initial Session

After nutrition referral

Obtain Referral Data
Site of treatment
Biochemical parameters
MD's goals—curative vs palliative
Medical history, including metastases, other disease diagnosis
Medication, including chemo, vitamins/minerals, herbs
Planned treatment, including surgery, chemotherapy, radiation
ADLs per Chemotherapy Toxicity Criteria

Initial Session

30-60 minutes

Assessment: Height, weight, usual body weight, % weight loss over time, lifestyle/psychosocial/nutrition history, history of side effects of treatment, smoking pattern.
Intervention: Self-management training: appropriate meal pattern, high-calorie/high-protein supplements; address other medical conditions, eg, diabetes, CAD. Mutually set goals.

For all patients receiving irradiation to any part of the GI tract or total body irradiation (TBI)

Communication: Summary to radiation oncologist. Documentation included in medical records. cc to medical oncologist/PCP.

First Follow-up Session

15-30 minutes

Assessment: % weight loss over time, food/supplement intakes, ADLs, side effects of treatment.
Intervention: Self-management training: increase intake of high-calorie/high-protein supplements, as needed; alternate feeding routes/administration as needed; skills to meet goals. Side effects may indicate need to change meds or diet. If so, discuss with oncologist.

All other patients

Communication: Summary to radiation oncologist. Documentation included in medical records. Long-term goals and plans for ongoing care stated. cc to medical oncologist/PCP.

Assessment: % weight loss over time, food/supplement intakes, ADLs, side effects of treatment.
Intervention: Self-management training: increase intake of high-calorie/high-protein supplements (if weight loss, alternative feeding routes/administration), skills to meet goals; side effects may indicate need to change meds. If so, discuss with oncologist.

Communication: Summary to radiation oncologist. Documentation included in medical records. Long-term goals and plans for ongoing care stated. cc to medical oncologist/PCP.

Ongoing Follow-up Session

15 minutes. GI or TBI irradiation patients (as needed).

Assessment: % weight loss over time, food/supplement intakes, ADLs, side effects of treatment.
Intervention: Self-management training: increase intake of high-calorie/high-protein supplements (if weight loss, skills to meet goals), side effects may indicate need to change meds. If so, discuss with oncologist.

PCP = primary care provider
PG-SGA = Patient-Generated
          Subjective Global Assessment

Medical Nutrition Therapy Across the Continuum of Care

©1998, The American Dietetic Association
Developed by ADA and Morrison Health Care.

Figure 3.3a Cancer (Medical) Session Process

CANCER (MEDICAL)
Medical Nutrition Therapy Protocol

Session/length: #1 for 60 minutes (referred to RD based on PG-SGA)

Session Process
Refer to Section II MNT Protocols for Implementation Guidelines.

Assessment
A. Obtain clinical data.
   1. Laboratory values with dates (within 15 days of session): albumin, prealbumin, electrolytes, BUN, creatinine, calcium, magnesium, phosphorus, LFT, glucose, CBC, ANC (if appropriate)
   2. Physician's goals for client treatment (eg, palliative or curative)
   3. Medical history: diabetes, cardiovascular disease, renal disease, GI abnormalities (ulcer, spastic bowel, reflux, etc), site of metastases (if any), prior surgery(s)
   4. Medications that affect nutrition therapy: antiemetics, antidiarrheals, steroids, antibiotics
   5. Treatment: chemotherapy: specific drugs and cycle; radiation: specific site
   6. ADLs and performance status: Chemotherapy Toxicity Criteria
   7. Clinical signs and symptoms: Chemotherapy Toxicity Criteria

B. Interview client/caregiver.
   1. Clinical data: current height/weight, calculate BMI, % weight loss over time, usual body weight
   2. Nutrition history: usual food intake, calculate current intake of calories and protein, weight history, use of vitamin/mineral/herb supplement(s), over-the-counter drugs, use of alcohol and tobacco pattern (if applicable)
   3. Exercise pattern: type of activity and duration
   4. Psychosocial and economic issues: living situation, cooking facilities, finances, educational background, literacy, employment, ethnic or religious belief considerations, family support, food assistance (if applicable)
   5. Knowledge/readiness to learn basic food/meal planning, attitude

Intervention
A. Provide self-management training of client on identified goals/nutrition prescription.
   1. Importance of adequate nutrition during cancer treatment
   2. Basic nutrition:
      • Cancer treatment vs cancer prevention eating guides (as applicable)
      • Weight management if needed for certain clients (eg, breast cancer, lymphoma)
   3. Calories and protein based on individual needs
   4. Calorie- and nutrient-dense foods/supplements
   5. Type of foods to decrease severity of side effects from treatment: texture, consistency, temperature, seasoning

Medical Nutrition Therapy Across the Continuum of Care

Figure 3.3a Cancer (Medical) Session Process (continued)

6. Potential food/drug interactions pertinent to client

7. Evaluation of medical nutrition supplements to provide appropriate nutrition vs calorie supplements

8. Evaluation of complementary nutrition treatment including diets, herbal preparations, megadoses of vitamins

9. Safe food handling practices

B. Provide self-management training and materials.
1. Review education materials containing information on (as needed for specific symptom management)
   - High-calorie, high-protein diet
   - Food Pyramid
   - Clear liquid diet
   - Lactose-controlled diet
   - Low-residue diet
   - Modification in texture
   - High-fiber diet
   - Neutropenic precautions
   - Food/drug interaction guidelines
2. *Outcome Measurements*
   - Meets goal(s) set with dietitian, eg, 6 small meals or snacks a day and increase protein intake through snacks.
   - Verbalizes potential food/drug interaction.
   - Chemotherapy Toxicity Criteria evaluation
3. Document on Initial Assessment Form and Nutrition Progress Notes.

C. Follow up
1. Schedule appointment as identified from PG-SGA.
2. *Expected Outcomes*
   - Maintains weight and nutritional status by changing dietary intake as needed.
   - Adopts individualized eating plan.
   - Improves functional status and ADLs.
   - Improves tolerance of foods.

Communication
1. Instruct client/caregiver to call with questions/concerns.
2. Place Initial Assessment and Nutrition Progress Notes in client's medical record. Send copy to PCP.
3. Discuss notes with oncologist and/or health care team members as needed.
4. Schedule appointment with client/oncologist/RD to discuss alternative route for nutrition as needed.

Figure 3.3a Cancer (Medical) Session Process (continued)

CANCER (MEDICAL)
Medical Nutrition Therapy Protocol

Session/length: #2, 3 for 15-30 minutes

Session Process

Assessment
Clinical data collected
- Current weight and % change since last session
- Current diet and supplementation use
- Biochemical data as available
- Functional status: ADLs
- Current medications
- Current treatment plan

Outcome Measurements: change in client's
- Weight
- Food intake record
- Laboratory values
- ADLs per Chemotherapy Toxicity Criteria
- Chemotherapy Toxicity Criteria
- Medications

Intervention
A. Adjust goals/nutrition prescription
   Review records, evaluate client's adherence and understanding, and provide feedback on food/meal planning.
   - Calories
   - Protein
   - ADLs

B. Provide self-management training and materials
   1. Change in client's status: weight and laboratory values, changes as appropriate
   2. Alternative route of nutrition support, if applicable. If weight loss >10%, discuss possible use of tube feeding and administration of tube feeding.
   3. Review education materials containing information on
      - Diet changes
      - Supplements, as needed
      - Recipe ideas
      - Potential food/drug interaction

Figure 3.3a Cancer (Medical) Session Process (continued)

4. *Expected Outcomes*
   - Maintains weight or minimizes weight loss.
   - Replenishes or preserves nutrition parameters.
   - Verbalizes food/drug interaction.
   - Adopts individualized healthy eating plan.

5. Document on Nutrition Progress Notes.

C. Follow up
   Schedule appointment as indicated from PG-SGA.

Communication
1. Instruct client/caregiver to call with questions/concerns.
2. Place Nutrition Progress Notes in client's medical record. Send copy to PCP.
3. Discuss notes with oncologist and/or health care team members as needed.
4. Schedule appointment with client/oncologist/RD to discuss alternative route for nutrition as needed.

Figure 3.3b Cancer (Radiation Oncology) Session Process

CANCER (RADIATION ONCOLOGY)

Medical Nutrition Therapy Protocol

Session/length: #1 for 30-60 minutes (referred to RD based on PG-SGA)

Session Process
Refer to Section II MNT Protocols for Implementation Guidelines.

Assessment

A. Obtain clinical data
   1. Physician's goals for client (eg, palliative or curative)
   2. Medical history: diabetes, cardiovascular disease, renal disease, GI abnormalities (ulcer, spastic bowel, reflux, etc), site of metastases (if any), prior surgerys
   3. Medications that affect nutrition therapy: antiemetics, antidiarrheals, steroids, antibiotics
   4. Treatment: radiation: specific site
   5. Performance status and ADLs: Chemotherapy Toxicity Criteria
   6. Clinical signs and symptoms: Chemotherapy Toxicity Criteria

B. Interview client/caregiver
   1. Clinical data: current height and weight, calculate BMI, % weight loss over time, usual body weight
   2. Nutrition history: usual food intake, calculate current intake of calories and protein, weight history, use of vitamin/mineral/herb supplement(s), over-the-counter drugs, use of alcohol and smoking pattern (if applicable)
   3. Exercise pattern: type of activity and duration
   4. Psychosocial and economic issues: living situation, cooking facilities, finances, educational background, literacy, employment, ethnic or religious belief considerations, family support, food assistance (if applicable)
   5. Knowledge/readiness to learn basic food/meal planning, attitude

Intervention

A. Provide self-management training of client on identified goals/nutrition prescription.
   1. Importance of adequate nutrition during cancer treatment
   2. Basic nutrition:
       • Cancer treatment vs cancer prevention eating guides (as applicable)
       • Weight management if needed for certain clients (eg, breast cancer, lymphoma)
   3. Calories and protein based on individual needs
   4. Calorie- and nutrient-dense foods/supplements
   5. Type of foods to decrease severity of side effects from treatment: texture, consistency, temperature, seasoning
   6. Potential food/drug interactions pertinent to client

Medical Nutrition Therapy Across the Continuum of Care

Figure 3.3b Cancer (Radiation Oncology) Session Process (continued)

7. Evaluation of medical nutrition supplements to provide appropriate nutrition vs calorie supplements
8. Evaluation of complementary nutrition treatment including diets, herbal preparations, megadoses of vitamins
9. Safe food handling practices

B. Provide self-management training and material
   1. Review education materials containing information on (as needed for specific symptom management)
      • High-calorie, high-protein foods
      • Food Pyramid
      • Clear liquid diet
      • Lactose-controlled diet
      • Low-residue diet
      • Modification in texture
      • High-fiber diet
      • Food/drug interaction guidelines
      • Neutropenic precautions
   2. *Outcome Measurements*
      • Meets goal(s) set with dietitian, eg, 6 small meals or snacks a day, and increase protein intake through snacks.
      • Verbalizes potential food/drug interaction.
   3. Document on Initial Assessment Form and Nutrition Progress Notes.

C. Follow up
   1. Schedule appointment as identified from PG-SGA.
   2. *Expected Outcomes*
      • Maintains weight and nutritional status by changing dietary intake as needed.
      • Adopts an individualized eating plan.

Communication
   1. Instruct client/caregiver to call with questions/concerns
   2. Place Initial Assessment and Nutrition Progress Notes in client's medical record
   3. Discuss notes with oncologist and/or health care team members as needed
   4. Schedule appointment with client/oncologist/RD to discuss alternative route for nutrition as needed

Medical Nutrition Therapy Across the Continuum of Care

Figure 3.3b Cancer (Radiation Oncology) Session Process (continued)

CANCER (RADIATION ONCOLOGY)
Medical Nutrition Therapy Protocol

Session/length: #2, 3 for 15-30 minutes

Session Process

Assessment
Clinical data collected
- Current weight and % change since last session
- Current diet and supplementation use
- Biochemical data as available
- Current ADLs/Chemotherapy Toxicity Criteria
- Current medications
- Chemotherapy Toxicity Criteria

Outcome Measurements: change in client's status
- Weight
- Food intake record
- Laboratory values
- ADLs per Chemotherapy Toxicity Criteria
- Medications

Intervention
A. Adjust goals/nutrition prescription
   Review records, evaluate client's adherence to program and understanding, and provide feedback on
   - Food/meal planning
   - Calories
   - Protein
   - ADLs

B. Provide counseling and education material
   1. Change in client's status: weight, laboratory values as appropriate
   2. Alternative route of nutrition support, if applicable. If weight loss >10%, discuss possible use of tube feeding and administration of tube feeding.
   3. Review education materials containing information on
      - Diet changes
      - Supplements, as needed
      - Recipe ideas
      - Potential food/drug interaction

Medical Nutrition Therapy Across the Continuum of Care

©1998, The American Dietetic Association
Developed by ADA and Morrison Health Care.

Figure 3.3b Cancer (Radiation Oncology) Session Process (continued)

4. *Expected Outcomes*
   * Maintains weight or minimizes weight loss.
   * Restores or preserves nutrition parameters.
   * Verbalizes food/drug interaction.
   * Adopts individualized eating plan.
5. Document on Nutrition Progress Notes.

E. Follow up
    Schedule appointment as indicated from PG-SGA.

Communication

1. Instruct client/caregiver to call with questions/concerns.
2. Place Nutrition Progress Notes in client's medical record.
3. Discuss notes with oncologist and/or health care team members as needed.
4. Schedule appointment with client/oncologist/RD to discuss alternative route for nutrition as needed.

Figure 3.4a Cancer (Medical) Nutrition Process

NUTRITION PROGRESS NOTES

Cancer (Medical)

Other Diagnosis:_____

Client's Name:
Phone Number:_____
Medical Record #:_____
DOB:_____ Gender:_____
Ethnic Background (Optional):_____
Referring Physician:_____

Outcomes of Medical Nutrition Therapy (MNT)

Expected outcome	Intervention provided to meet goal (Intervention = self-management training plus client verbalizes/ demonstrates)			Goal reached (√ indicates goal reached)		
Session	1 (60 min)	2 (30 min)	3 (30 min)	Date:___ 1	Date:___ 2	Date:___ 3
Clinical Outcomes				*Value*	*Value*	*Value*
Albumin (g/dL)				___	___	___
Prealbumin (mg/dL)				___	___	___
HgB (g/dL)				___	___	___
Hct (vol %)				___	___	___
Other _____				___	___	___
_____				___	___	___
_____				___	___	___
_____				___	___	___
Height____ Weight____				___	___	___
BMI____ UBW____				___ lb	___ lb	___ lb
Functional Outcome Chemotherapy Toxicity Criteria • ADLs ⇑ of ⇓						
MNT Goal____kcal____g Pro • Maintain adequate intake of kilo-calories and protein • Select foods to limit side effects	initial estimate __kcal _ g Pro			% of goal ___kcal _ g Pro	% of goal ___kcal _ g Pro	% of goal ___kcal _ g Pro
Behavioral Outcomes • Verbalizes importance of appropriate nutrition • Consumes high-calorie/protein foods • Consumes/avoids foods that lessen side effects of treatment • Avoids foods that may cause side effects with treatment • Uses appropriate/safe complementary nutrition therapies • Uses acceptable alternative feeding routes, such as enteral feedings, if oral intake not adequate • Uses appropriate supplements as needed • Adopts healthy eating plan *Overall Compliance Potential** • Comprehension • Receptivity • Adherence				E G P E G P E G P	E G P E G P E G P	E G P E G P E G P

Intervention: D Discussed, **R** Reinforced/Reviewed, ≠ Not reviewed, ˛ Outcome achieved, **N/A** Not applicable
*Compliance Potential: E - Excellent, **G** - Good, **P** - Poor

Date:_____
Comments:_____

_____
_____

Medical Nutrition Therapy Across the Continuum of Care

Figure 3.4a Cancer (Medical) Nutrition Process (continued)

Client Goals:____

Material Provided:____

Next Visit:____**RD**

Signature/Date

Date:_________

Comments:____

Client Goals:____

Material Provided:____

Next Visit:____**RD**

Signature/Date

Date:_________

Comments:____

Client Goals:____

Material Provided:____

Next Visit:____**RD**

Signature/Date

Medical Nutrition Therapy Across the Continuum of Care

Figure 3.4b Cancer (Radiation Oncology) Nutrition Process

NUTRITION PROGRESS NOTES
Cancer (Radiation Oncology)

Other Diagnosis: _____

Client's Name: _____
Phone Number: _____
Medical Record #: _____
DOB: _____ Gender: _____
Ethnic Background (Optional): _____
Referring Physician: _____

Outcomes of Medical Nutrition Therapy (MNT)

Expected outcome	Intervention provided to meet goal (Intervention = education plus client verbalizes/demonstrates)			Goal reached (√ indicates goal reached)		
Session	1 (60 min)	2 (30 min)	3 (30 min)	Date: _____ 1	Date: _____ 2	Date: _____ 3
Clinical Outcomes Blood pressure Height ____ Weight ____ BMI ____ UBW ____				*Value* __/__ ____ lb	*Value* __/__ ____ lb	*Value* __/__ ____ lb
Functional Outcome Chemotherapy Toxicity Criteria • ADLs ⇑ or ⇓						
MNT Goal ____ kcal ____ g Pro • Maintain adequate intake of kilo-calories and protein • Select foods to alleviate side effects of treatment	initial est. __kcal __g Pro			% of goal ___kcal ___g Pro	% of goal ___kcal ___g Pro	% of goal ___kcal ___g Pro
Behavioral Outcomes • Verbalizes importance of adequate nutrition • Consumes adequate calories to meet expected weight and maintain goal • Maintains hydration status as measured by blood pressure within normal limits, good skin turgor, no signs of dehydration or dizziness • Consumes high-kcal, low-protein supplements, as needed • Consumes/avoids foods that lessen side effects of treatment • Uses acceptable/safe complementary nutrition therapy • Accepts/utilizes alternative feeding routes (eg, tube feedings) to meet calorie/protein needs • Adopts healthy eating plan						
Overall Compliance Potential • Comprehension • Receptivity • Adherence				E G P E G P E G P	E G P E G P E G P	E G P E G P E G P

Intervention: D Discussed, R Reinforced/Reviewed, ≠ Not reviewed, √ Outcome achieved, N/A Not applicable
***Compliance Potential: E Excellent, G Good, P Poor**

Figure 3.4b Cancer (Radiation Oncology) Nutrition Process (continued)

Date:_____

Comments:_____
_____
_____
_____
_____

Client Goals:_____
Material Provided:_____

Next Visit:_____RD
                                        Signature/Date

Date:_____

Comments:_____
_____
_____
_____
_____

Client Goals:_____
Material Provided:_____

Next Visit:_____RD
                                        Signature/Date

Date:_____

Comments:_____
_____
_____
_____
_____

Client Goals:_____
Material Provided:_____

Next Visit:_____RD
                                        Signature/Date

Medical Nutrition Therapy Across the Continuum of Care

Figure 3.5 Bibliography

Bibliography

Assessing the Nutritional Status of Dialysis Clients Using Subjective Global Assessment. 5K9512. Chicago: Baxter Healthcare Corporation; 1993. (For additional information on SGA.)

Bloch AS. *Nutrition Management of the Cancer Patient.* Rockville, Md: Aspen Publishers, Inc; 1990.

Detsky AS, Baker JP, O'Rourke K, Johnston N, Whittwell J, Mendelson RA, Jeejeebhoy KN. et al. Predicting nutrition-associated complications for clients undergoing gastrointestinal surgery. *JPEN.* 1987;11:440-446.

Detsky AS, McLaughlin JR, Baker JP, Johnston N, Whittaker S, Mendelson RA, Jeejeebhoy KN. What is subjective global assessment of nutritional status? *JPEN.* 1987;11:8-13.

Detsky AS, Smalley PS, Chang J. Is this patient malnourished? *JAMA.* 1994;271(1):54-57.

Enia G, Sicuso C, Alati G, Zoccali C. Subjective global assessment of nutrition in dialysis clients. *Nephrol Dial Transplant.* 1993;8(10):1094-1098.

Garrell DR, Jobin N, deJonge LHM. Should we still use the Harris-Benedict Equations? *Nutr Clin Prac.* 1996;11(3):99-103.

Hunter AMB. Nutrition management of patients with neoplastic disease of the head and neck treated with radiation therapy. Nutr Clin Prac. 1996;11:157-169.

Manning EM, Shenkin A. Nutrition assessment in the critically ill. *Crit Care Clinics.* 1995;11(3):91-100.

McMahon K, Decker G, Ottery FO. Integrating proactive nutritional assessment in clinical practices to prevent complications and cost. *Seminars in Oncology.* 1998;24(2):20-27.

Nagel MR. Nutrition screening: identifying patients at risk for malnutrition. *Nutr Clin Prac.* 1993;8(4):171-175.

Nixon DW. *The Cancer Recovery Eating Plan.* New York: Times Books; 1994.

Oken MM, Creech RH, Tormey DC, Horton J, Davis T, McFadden ET, Carbone PP. Toxicity and response criteria of the Eastern Cooperative Oncology Group. *Am J Clin Oncol.* 1992;5:649-655.

Figure 3.5 Bibliography (continued)

Ottery FD. Algorithm of optimal nutritional intervention. *Nutr Oncol.* 1994;1(2):7.

Ottery FD. Oncology client-generated SGA of nutritional status. *Nutr Oncol.* 1994;1(2):9.

Ottery FD, DeBolt S, Kasenic S, Wilby M, Castaneda-Mendez K. *Protocol 9601: Validation of Nutritional Triage Using the Scored Patient-Generated Subjective Global Assessment (PG-SGA).* Philadelphia: Society for Nutritional Oncology Adjuvant Therapy; 1996. For copy, send e-mail request to noatpres@pol.net.

Ottery FD. Supportive nutrition to prevent cachexia and improve quality of life. *Semin Oncol.* 1995;22(suppl 3):98S.

Ottery FD. Modification of subjective global assessment (SGA) of nutritional status for oncology patients. Paper presented at 19th Clinical Congress, American Society for Parenteral and Enteral Nutrition, Miami, Florida, January 15-18, 1995.

Wittes RE. *Manual of Oncologic Therapeutics.* Philadelphia: Lippincott; 1989:627-632.

Other Resources

ECOG (Eastern Cooperative Oncology Group), 303 Boylston Street, Brookline, Mass 02146-7648.

News release. Lewin Study results. ADA Web site at http://www.eatright.org/adamnt.html.

Gallagher AC, Coble-Voss A, Gussler JD, eds. *Nutrition Intervention and Patient Outcomes: A Self Study Manual.* Columbus, Ohio: Ross Products Division, Abbott Laboratories; 1995.

4

Calorie, Protein, Fluid, and Micronutrient Requirements

Cathy Martin, MS, RD, CNSD

Malnutrition is common among cancer patients. Physiological changes seen in the cancer patient include protein catabolism, muscle wasting, and immune compromise (see Chapter 6, *Changes in Carbohydrate, Protein, and Fat Metabolism in Cancer*). Early nutrition intervention and provision of adequate energy, protein, fluid, vitamins, minerals, and trace elements is necessary to prevent further catabolism, nutrient deficiencies, and to replete nutrition stores. Factors that influence the nutrition status of the cancer patient include 1) physiologic abnormalities related to the tumor itself, host response to the tumor, or the impact of antineoplastic treatment and potential side effects and 2) mechanical issues such as the tumor size and location. Inadequate intake and utilization of nutrients may be the result of cancer treatment, anorexia, malabsorption, obstruction, or metabolic alterations that increase specific nutrient requirements (1). Inadequate nutrient intake contributes to weight loss and may result in decreased response rates to antineoplastic therapy, decreased performance status, and decreased survival (2).

Energy Requirements

Energy requirements for patients with cancer cannot be generalized. Studies addressing energy requirements specific to tumor type or location in humans have provided limited data and considerable variability (3). Energy requirements in cancer patients span the spectrum of hypermetabolic (~25%), eumetabolic, and hypometabolic (~30%). Alterations in metabolism are likely due to body composition, state of malnutrition, tumor type, and disease stage (3,4,5,6,7). Problems exist in interpreting available data which address energy requirements in cancer patients. This stems from the fact that much of the data is from animal models, where tumor burden is often a large part of body weight and cell turnover is generally more rapid than it is in humans. Individual energy needs are most often estimated using standard or factorial methods (Table 4.1).

Table 4.1   Quick Guide to Estimating Energy Needs in Adults (4,5,8,9,10,11,12)

These equations are useful as initial estimates of energy needs. Energy needs should be adjusted as the patient's nutritional status changes. Actual (current) body weight is used; however, it is recommended that ideal body weight (IBW) be used in obese patients (>120% IBW), because adjusted body weight for obesity has not been validated (10,16,17).

20 kcal/kg	Initial re-feeding of malnourished/depleted patient
21–25 kcal/kg	Obese patients for maintenance
25–30 kcal/kg	Maintenance/standard
30–35 kcal/kg	Malnourished and/or extensive treatment (see Chapter 2, *Patient-Generated Subjective Global Assessment*)/ bone marrow transplant
35–45 kcal/kg	Depleted and/or hypermetabolic

Energy requirements must be individualized and evaluated based on the current clinical issues. Cancer patients in the intensive care unit may require more precise estimation of energy needs by indirect calorimetry (Exhibit 4.1).

Exhibit 4.1   Methods of Estimating Energy Needs in Adults

These equations are useful as initial estimates of energy needs. Energy needs should be adjusted as the patient's nutritional status changes. Actual (current) body weight is used; however, it is recommended that ideal body weight (IBW) be used in obese patients (>120% IBW), because adjusted body weight for obesity has not been validated (10,16,17).

Factorial Methods/Predictive Equations
Harris-Benedict (4,12,14,18)
BEE = Basal Energy Expenditure
BEE (men) = 66.47 + 13.75 (wt in kg) + 5 (ht in cm) − 6.76 (age in yrs)
BEE (women) = 655.1 + 9.56 (wt in kg) + 1.85 (ht in cm) − 4.68 (age in yrs)
EEE (Estimated Energy Expenditure) = BEE × activity factor (AF) × injury factor (IF)

Activity factors	1.2	= bed
	1.3	= ambulatory
Injury factors	1.2–1.3	= minor surgery and cancer treatment
	1.4	= major surgery or hypermetabolic/BMT (bone marrow transplant)

(See Chapter 9, *MNT in Bone Marrow Transplantation,* for injury factors specific to BMT.)

Use: Most common; recommend BEE × 1.3–1.5 for most cancer patients
Pro: Inexpensive; accuracy improves as method repeated
Con: Not as accurate as indirect methods; may overestimate needs
Required equipment: None

Indirect Methods
Indirect Calorimetry (5,10,14,15,17,19,20,21)
REE = Resting Energy Expenditure
REE = (3.9 (VO_2)) + 1.1 (VCO_2) × 1.44
    VO_2 = oxygen consumption
    VCO_2 = carbon dioxide production
EEE = REE × 1.1 (stressed/maintenance)
    REE × 1.3 (repletion)
RQ = (VCO_2/VO_2) = respiratory quotient as a measure of substrate utilization
    RQ > 1.0 (suggests need to decrease total calories, likely result of overfeeding)
    RQ = 1.0 (carbohydrate oxidation)
    RQ = 0.85 (mixed substrate oxidation = preferred RQ)
    RQ = 0.8 (protein oxidation)
    RQ = 0.7 (fat oxidation)
Use: Critical care setting, ventilatory dependent patient, obese, severely malnourished, severely stressed, patients with questionable dry weight
Pro: Accurate
Con: Costly; patients with FIO_2* > 50% for adequate oxygenation, or chronic obstructive pulmonary disease**
Required equipment: Metabolic-cart-trained clinician

Key: *FIO_2 = fraction of inspired oxygen
    **COPD

Provision of mixed caloric substrate, both carbohydrate and fat, is necessary to prevent further protein breakdown in the cancer patient (Table 4.2). Overfeeding, via provision of excess calories, must be avoided, as it may lead to respiratory compromise and decreased immune response (5,13,14,15).

Table 4.2   Distribution of Macronutrient Provision in Adults

Substrates	Provision as % of Total Calories
Carbohydrate (4,8,15)	30%–70%
Fat (4,8,15)	20%–50%
	Higher levels maybe needed in patients with hyperglycemia or to ensure adequate caloric intake.
	Minimum of 4%–10% to prevent essential fatty acid deficiency/linoleic acid
Protein (4,9,15)	15%–25%

Protein Requirements in Cancer Patients

Upon clinical or laboratory evaluation of the cancer patient, there is often evidence of protein malnutrition as wasting of lean body mass or abnormalities of serum transport proteins such as albumin, transferrin, or prealbumin (see Chapter 2, *Patient-Generated Subjective Global Assessment*). Positive nitrogen balance is necessary to optimize the chances of maintaining lean body mass and immune competence. Loss of lean tissue can contribute significantly to weakness, fatigue, and increase risk of complications such as decubiti, infection, poor tolerance to treatment modalities, inability to wean from ventilator dependence, poor wound healing, immune compromise, and pulmonary emboli due to deep vein thrombosis. While normal requirements of protein, in terms of calorie to nitrogen ratio, are in the range of 125:1 to 150:1, a more appropriate ratio for malnourished patients is 100:1 (4,9). Septic patients may even approach 80:1. Nitrogen balance may be utilized, but the test is impractical for the majority of cancer patients. It is generally easier and more efficient to calculate protein requirements using grams of protein per kilogram of actual body weight (see Table 4.3).

Table 4.3   Quick Guide to Estimating Protein Needs in Adults (4,8,12,22,23)

Protein Needs	Condition
0.5–0.8 g/kg	Hepatic or renal compromise including BUN (Blood Urea Nitrogen) approaching 100 mg/dL or rising ammonia levels
0.8–1.0 g/kg	RDA for adults
1.0–1.5 g/kg	Most cancer patients Use lower or higher end based on visceral protein status
1.5 g/kg	Bone marrow transplant patients
1.5–2.0 g/kg	Depleted cancer patient

Notes: Use actual (current) body weight. May use ideal body weight (IBW) in obese patients (>120%IBW).

Fluid Requirements in Cancer Patients

Fluid status must be monitored routinely in the cancer patient, especially in those undergoing surgery, chemotherapy, or radiation, as treatment methods may contribute to alterations in fluid status. Weight, intake and output, and laboratory data are appropriate measures to utilize in daily assessing hydration status (see Chapter 11, *Enteral Nutrition in Adult Medical/Surgical Oncology* and Chapter 12, *Parenteral Nutrition in Adult Medical/Surgical Oncology*). Fluid needs vary depending on the current condition of the patient and the environment. Fluid may be provided enterally (oral or tube fed) via intake of water, beverages, and foodstuffs, or parenterally. Electrolyte and fluid replacement is common when patients have the following: anorexia, excessive diarrhea, fever, sweating, dehydration, wound dehiscence (a bursting open), decubitus ulcers, gastrointestinal losses, renal losses, hypermetabolism, or hyperventilation (9,12). Adequate hydration in the presence of cardiac, respiratory, or renal dysfunction is challenging and requires prudent management; fluid restrictions may be necessary. Careful attention must also be paid to potential overhydration of patients receiving multiple intravenous fluids, chemotherapy agents, and other medications. The simplest method for estimating fluid needs is based on caloric intake and the most precise is based on body surface area (Table 4.4).

Table 4.4   Estimating Fluid Needs in Adults with Normal Renal and Hepatic Function (8,9,22,24)

Method		Guideline
RDA/Caloric Intake-Based		1 mL/kcal
Age-based	<55 yrs of age	30–40 mL/kg
	55–65 yrs of age	30 mL/kg
	>65 yrs of age	25 mL/kg
Weight-based		0.5 oz/lb (15 mL/lb) of IBW
Body Surface Area (BSA)		Fluid needs (mL) = BSA × 1500
		Fluid needs (L) = BSA × 1.5
$BSA\ (m^2) = \sqrt{\dfrac{weight\ (kg) \times height\ (cm)}{60}}$		

Notes: Use actual (current) body weight. May use ideal body weight (IBW) in obese patients (>120% IBW).

Micronutrient Requirements

Vitamins, minerals, and trace elements are known to play an important and necessary role in normal maintenance of the body. When inadequate ingestion of these micronutrients occurs, deficiencies may result. The cancer patient may be at increased risk for micronutrient deficiencies due to anorexia, cachexia, malnutrition, effects of cancer therapy, tumor type, malabsorption, and/or metabolic or gastrointestinal alterations (25,26). Supplementation is appropriate to replete these patients' micronutrient status. Cancer patients undergoing chemotherapy (Chapter 6, *Chemotherapy and Nutrition Implications*), radiation (Chapter 7, *Nutrition Implications with the Radiation Therapy Patient*), or surgery (Chapter 8, *Nutrition Implications of Surgical Oncology*) may have increased losses or diminished absorptive capacity due to the specific site receiving treatment, surgical impact, or chemotherapeutic agent used (Table 4.5).

Table 4.5   Absorption Sites in the Gastrointestinal Tract (11,22,25)

Site	Vitamin, Mineral, Electrolytes
Duodenum	Calcium, magnesium, iron, chloride
Jejunum	Vitamin C, thiamine (B1), riboflavin (B2), pyridoxine (B6). folic acid, water soluble vitamins
Ileum	Vitamins B_{12}, A, D, E, K
Colon	Sodium, potassium, water

The role of micronutrients and their relationship to the immune system in humans is not well documented to date. Current research is focused on the role of micronutrients in cancer prevention (26). (See also Table 12.1, Chapter 12, *Parenteral Nutrition in Medical/Surgical Oncology*.) The RDAs offer recommendations for safe and adequate minimum daily intakes of micronutrients (22). Enteral and parenteral dosing recommendations do differ (Tables 4.6, 4.7, 4.8). The optimal level for maximal health benefit has not yet been established for the cancer patient, but megadosing should be avoided. Future studies may enlighten clinicians as to whether or not cancer patients have specific altered micronutrient requirements.

Dietary Reference Intakes (DRIs) provide quantitative estimates of nutrient intakes to be used for planning and assessing diets for healthy people. The DRIs replace and expand more precisely the series of Recommended Dietary Allowances (RDAs) that have been published since 1941 by the Food and Nutrition Board. In addition to including RDAs as goals for intake by individuals, the DRIs consist of three new types of reference values: the Adequate Intake (AI), the Tolerable Upper Level (UL), and the Estimated Average Requirement (EAR). The Adequate Intake (AI) is a level judged to meet the needs of all individuals in a group and is used when an RDA cannot be determined. The Tolerable Upper Level (UL) represents the highest level of daily nutrient intake that will have no risks of adverse health effects to almost all individuals in the general population. The Estimated Average Requirement (EAR) is a nutrient intake value that is estimated to meet the requirement of half the healthy individuals in a group. The newest recommendations based on the DRIs include calcium, phosphorus, Vitamin D, magnesium, and fluoride in addition to most recently, folate, choline, and the B vitamins. Dietitians should be aware that more updates are coming in the future (31).

Table 4.6 Recommended Dietary Allowances (22)

Category	Age (years) or condition	Weight[b] (kg)	Weight[b] (lb)	Height[b] (cm)	Height[b] (in)	Protein (g)	Fat-Soluble Vitamins — Vitamin A (µg RE)[c]	Vitamin D (µg)[d]	Vitamin E (mg α-TE)[e]	Vitamin K (µg)	Water-Soluble Vitamins — Vitamin C (mg)	Thiamin (mg)	Riboflavin (mg)	Niacin (mg NE)[f]	Vitamin B_6 (mg)	Folate (µg)	Vitamin B_{12} (µg)	Minerals — Calcium (mg)	Phosphorus (mg)	Magnesium (mg)	Iron (mg)	Zinc (mg)	Iodine (µg)	Selenium (µg)
Infants	0.0–0.5	6	13	60	24	13	375	7.5	3	5	30	0.3	0.4	5	0.3	25	0.3	400	300	40	6	5	40	10
	0.5–1.0	9	20	71	28	14	375	10	4	10	35	0.4	0.5	6	0.6	35	0.5	600	500	60	10	5	50	15
Children	1–3	13	29	90	35	16	400	10	6	15	40	0.7	0.8	9	1.0	50	0.7	800	800	80	10	10	70	20
	4–6	20	44	112	44	24	500	10	7	20	45	0.9	1.1	12	1.1	75	1.0	800	800	120	10	10	90	20
	7–10	28	62	132	52	28	700	10	7	30	45	1.0	1.2	13	1.4	100	1.4	800	800	170	10	10	120	30
Males	11–14	45	99	157	62	45	1000	10	10	45	50	1.3	1.5	17	1.7	150	2.0	1200	1200	270	12	15	150	40
	15–18	66	145	176	69	59	1000	10	10	65	60	1.5	1.8	20	2.0	200	2.0	1200	1200	400	12	15	150	50
	19–24	72	160	177	70	58	1000	10	10	70	60	1.5	1.7	19	2.0	200	2.0	1200	1200	350	10	15	150	70
	25–50	79	174	176	70	63	1000	5	10	80	60	1.5	1.7	19	2.0	200	2.0	800	800	350	10	15	150	70
	51+	77	170	173	68	63	1000	5	10	80	60	1.2	1.4	15	2.0	200	2.0	800	800	350	10	15	150	70
Females	11–14	46	101	157	62	46	800	10	8	45	50	1.1	1.3	15	1.4	150	2.0	1200	1200	280	15	12	150	45
	15–18	55	120	163	64	44	800	10	8	55	60	1.1	1.3	15	1.5	180	2.0	1200	1200	300	15	12	150	50
	19–24	58	128	164	65	46	800	10	8	60	60	1.1	1.3	15	1.6	180	2.0	1200	1200	280	15	12	150	55
	25–50	63	138	163	64	50	800	5	8	65	60	1.1	1.3	15	1.6	180	2.0	800	800	280	15	12	150	55
	31+	65	143	160	63	50	800	5	8	65	60	1.0	1.2	13	1.6	180	2.0	800	800	280	10	12	150	55
Pregnant						60	800	10	10	65	70	1.5	1.6	17	2.2	400	2.2	1200	1200	320	30	15	175	65
Lactating	1st 6 months					65	1300	10	12	65	95	1.6	1.8	20	2.1	280	2.6	1200	1200	355	15	19	200	75
	2nd 6 months					62	1200	10	11	65	90	1.6	1.7	20	2.1	260	2.6	1200	1200	340	15	16	200	73

Reprinted with permission from *Recommended Dietary Allowances*, 10th ed. ©1989 by The National Academy of Sciences. Courtesy of The National Academy Press, Washington, D.C.

[a]The allowances, expressed as average daily intakes over time, are intended to provide for individual variations among most normal persons as they live in the United States under usual environmental stresses. Diets should be based on a variety of common foods in order to provide other nutrients for which human requirements have bee less well defined.

[b]Weights and heights of Reference Adults are actual medians for the U.S. population of the disgnated ages, as reported by NHANES II. The use of these figures does not imply that the height-to-weight ratios are ideal.

[c]Retinol equivalents. 1 retinol equivalent = 1 µg retinol or 6 µg β-carotene.

[d]As cholecalciferol. 10 µg cholecalciferol = 400 ɪᴜ of vitamin D.

[e]α-Tocopherol equivalents. 1 mg d-α tocopherol = 1 α-ᴛᴇ. See text for variation in allowances and calculation of vitamin E activity of the diet as α-tocopherol equivalents.

[f]1 ɴᴇ (niacin equivalent) is equal to 1 mg of niacin or 60 mg of dietary tryptophan.

Table 4.7   Estimated Safe and Adequate Daily Dietary Intakes of Selected Vitamins and Minerals[a] (22)

Category	Age (years)	Vitamins	
		Biotin (µg)	Pantothenic Acid (mg)
Infants	0–0.5	10	2
	0.5–1	15	3
Children and adolescents	1–3	20	3
	4–6	25	3–4
	7–10	30	4–5
	11+	30–100	4–7
Adults		30–100	4–7

Category	Age (years)	Trace Elements[b]				
		Copper (mg)	Manganese (mg)	Fluoride (mg)	Chromium (µg)	Molybdenum (µg)
Infants	0–0.5	0.4–0.6	0.3–0.6	0.1–0.5	10-40	15-30
	0.5-1	0.6-0.7	0.6-1.0	0.2-1.0	20-60	20-40
Children and adolescents	1-3	0.7-1.0	1.0-1.5	0.5-1.5	20-80	25-50
	4-6	1.0-1.5	1.5-2.0	1.0-2.5	30-120	30-75
	7-10	1.0-2.0	2.0-3.0	1.5-2.5	50-200	50-150
	11+	1.5-2.5	2.0-5.0	1.5-2.5	50-200	75-250
Adults		1.5-3.0	2.0-5.0	1.5-4.0	50-200	75-250

[a]Because there is less information on which to base allowances, these figures are not given in the main table of RDA and are provided here in the form of ranges of recommended intakes.
[b]Since the toxic levels for many trace elements may be only several times usual intakes, the upper leves for the trace elements given in this table should not be habitually exceeded.

Reprinted with permission from *Recommended Dietary Allowances,* 10th ed. ©1989 by The National Academy of Sciences. Courtesy of The National Academy Press, Washington, D.C.

Table 4.8   American Medical Association: IV Vitamins and Trace Elements (27)

Vitamin	RDA	Intravenous Multivitamin (IV)	Intramuscular Multivitamin, water soluble (IM)
A (IU)	4000–5000[a]	3300	—
D (IU)	400	200	—
E (IU)	12–15	10	—
Ascorbic acid (mg)	45	100	100
Folacin (mcg)	400	400	400
Niacin (mg)	12–20	40	40
Riboflavin (mg)	1.1–1.8	3.6	3.6
Thiamin (mg)	1.0–1.5	3.0	3.0
B_6—Pyridoxine (mg)	1.6–2.0	4.0	4.0
B_{12}—Cyanocobalamin (mcg)	3.0	5.0	5.0
Pantothenic acid (mg)	5–10[b]	15.0	15.0
Biotin	150–300[b]	60.0	60.0

Reprinted with permission from *Recommended Dietary Allowances,* 10th ed. ©1989 by The National Academy of Sciences. Courtesy of The National Academy Press, Washington, D.C.

Refeeding Syndrome

Repletion or refeeding the malnourished cancer patient may create new and unique problems. Resulting complications known as the "refeeding syndrome" involve intracellular shifts of potassium, magnesium, phosphorus, and calcium, resulting in low serum levels. Gastrointestinal, respiratory, cardiac, and renal dysfunction may occur and are likely due to electrolyte imbalance (28). Close, continuous monitoring of electrolyte disturbances is required for a minimum of 5 to 7 days. Low serum levels of electrolytes, namely potassium, phosphorus, and magnesium, require appropriate replacement (see Chapter 6, *Chemotherapy and Nutrition Implications* and Chapter 12, *Parenteral Nutrition in Medical/Surgical*

Oncology). Hyperglycemia and fluid overload may occur with overfeeding or overhydration. Repleting the malnourished cancer patient should be initiated by providing less than 100% of energy needs (20 kcal/kg). Overfeeding must be avoided, so as not to increase the risk of "refeeding syndrome." After the patient is stabilized, energy needs may be increased as appropriate. Protein should be provided in adequate amounts to replete stores (1.2–1.5 g/kg). Further research may allow clinicians to better predict which cancer patients are more at risk for refeeding syndrome.

Summary

Malnutrition in the cancer patient can prove challenging to even the experienced clinician. It is important to remember when estimating energy, protein, fluid, and micronutrient requirements, that they are just that, estimates. Consequently, routine follow-up is necessary to determine whether estimated nutrient requirements are being met (orally, enterally, or parenterally). Provision of adequate nutrition is necessary to maintain or replete the cancer patient and individualized patient care is warranted. Caution must be taken to avoid overfeeding and further contributing to metabolic aberrations. The future may reveal specific immunomodulating nutrients of benefit to cancer patients. Specific nutrients may include glutamine, arginine, omega-3 fatty acids, vitamin A, vitamin C, vitamin E, zinc, and selenium, but to date, research has not demonstrated improved outcome with these nutrients in cancer patients (29). Enhanced patient tolerance to cancer therapy is the aim of adequate nutrition in the cancer patient.

References

1. Mercadante S. Nutrition in cancer patients. *Supp Care Cancer*. 1996;4:10–20.
2. Eastern Cooperative Oncology Group. Prognostic effect of weight loss prior to chemotherapy in cancer patients. *Am J Med*. 1980;69:491–497.
3. Fredrix E, Soeters P, Wouters E, et al. Effect of different tumor types on resting energy expenditure. *Cancer Research*. 1991;51:6138–6141.
4. Dempsey D, Mullen J. Macronutrient requirements in the malnourished cancer patient: How much of what and why? *Cancer*. 1985;55:290–294.
5. Merrick H, Long C, Grecos G, et al. Energy requirements for cancer patients and the effect of total parenteral nutrition. *JPEN J Parenter Enteral Nutr*. 1998;12(1):8–14.
6. Sakurai Y, Klein S. Metabolic alteration in patients with cancer: nutritional implications. *Surg Today*. 1998;28:247–257.
7. Mulligan K, Bloch A. Energy expenditure and protein metabolism in human immunodeficiency virus infection and cancer cachexia. *Sem in Oncol*. 1998;25(2:S6):82–91.
8. A Consensus Statement of the American College of Chest Physicians. Applied nutrition in ICU patients. *Chest*. 1997;111:769–778.
9. Harrison L, Brennan M. *Current Problems in Surgery*. Vol XXXII, no. 10. St Louis, Mo: Mosby-Year Book; 1995. (AU: page reference?)
10. Amato P, Keating K, Quercia R, et al. Formulaic methods of estimating caloric requirements in mechanically ventilated obese patients: A reappraisal. *Nutr Clin Prac*. 1995;10(6): 229–232.
11. *Dietitian's Handbook of Enteral and Parenteral Nutrition*. 2nd ed. Skipper A. Gaithersburg, Md: Aspen Publishers, Inc, 1998.
12. Herrmann V, Petruska P. Nutrition support in bone marrow transplant recipients. *Nutr Clin Prac*. 1993;8:19–27.
13. Talpers S, Romberger D, Bunce S, et al. Nutritionally associated increased carbon dioxide production: Excess total calories vs high proportion of carbohydrate calories. *Chest*. 1992;102:551–555.
14. Osborne B, Saba A, Wood S, et al. Clinical comparison of three methods to determine resting energy expenditure. *Nutr Clin Prac*. 1994;9(6):241–246.
15. Ireton-Jones C, Borman K, Turner W. Nutrition considerations in the management of ventilator-dependent patients. *Nutr ClinPrac*. 1993;8(2):60–64.

16. Ireton-Jones C, Turner W. Actual or ideal body weight: Which should be used to predict energy expenditure? *J Am Diet Assoc.* 1991;91:193–195.

17. Choban P, Burge J, Flancbaum L. Nutrition support of obese hospitalized patients. *Nutr Clin Prac.* 1997;12(4):149–154.

18. Garrel D, Jobin N, DeJonge L. Should we still use the Harris and Benedict equations? *Nutr Clin Prac.* 1996;11(3):99–103.

19. Long C, Schaffel N, Geiger J, et al. Metabolic response to injury and illness: Estimation of energy and protein needs from indirect calorimetry and nitrogen balance. *JPEN.* 1979;3:452–456.

20. Porter C, Cohen N. Indirect calorimetry in critically ill patients: Role of the clinical dietitian in interpreting results. *J Amer Diet Assoc.* 1996;96(1):49–57.

21. McClave S, Snider H. Use of indirect calorimetry in clinical nutrition. *Nutr Clin Prac.* 1992;7(5):207–221.

22. Food and Nutrition Board, Commission on Life Sciences, National Research Council. *Recommended Dietary Allowances.* 10th ed. Washington DC: National Academy Press; 1989.

23. Curtas S, Miles J, Klein J. Should protein be included in calorie calculations for a TPN prescription? *Nutr Clin Prac.* 1996;11(5):204–206.

24. Zeman F. Clinical *Nutrition and Dietetics.* New York: McMillan; 1991.

25. Grant J, Chapman G, Russell M. Malabsorption associated with surgical procedures and its treatment. *Nutr Clin Prac.* 1996;11(2):43–52.

26. Hoffman F. Micronutrient requirements in cancer patients. *Ca.* 1985;55:295–300.

27. American Medical Association Department of Foods and Nutrition. Multivitamin preparations for parenteral use: A statement by the Nutrition Advisory Group. *JPEN.* 1979;3(4):258–262.

28. Solomon S, Kirby D. The refeeding syndrome: A review. *JPEN.* 1990;14(1):90–97.

29. Klein S, Korentz R. Nutrition support in patients with cancer: What do the data really show? *Nutr Clin Prac.* 1994;9(3):91–100.

30. Yates, AA, Schlicker SA, Suitor CW. Dietary Reference Intakes: The new basis for recommendations for calcium and related nutrients, B vitamins, and choline. *J Am Diet Assoc.* 1998;98:699–706.

5

Changes in Carbohydrate, Protein, and Fat Metabolism in Cancer

Linda Nebeling, PhD, MPH, RD

The objective of this chapter is to present an overview of the relationship between nutrition and cancer as it relates to the initiation and promotion of tumor growth. A systematic review of the effects a tumor may have on normal carbohydrate, protein, and fat metabolism is described. Since the extent of disease varies across patients, not all metabolic alterations described will apply to every cancer patient. Issues related to nutrition and cancer treatment will be covered in other chapters and should be referred to when determining an appropriate care plan for the cancer patient.

Tumor Growth and Cachexia

The presence of a tumor may affect the patient's biochemical and metabolic functions, possibly leading to increased morbidity and mortality (1,2). Standard nutritional support may not always be effective in significantly improving the outcome in malnourished cancer patients due to changes in metabolism. The tumor, which is responsible for initiating these changes, can influence normal metabolism (3). Increased energy expenditure and elevations in basal metabolism, along with alterations in enzyme activity and the immune system occur in the patient (4). The end result is an alteration in energy requirements, carbohydrate, lipid, and protein metabolism (Table 5.1). Additional alterations can be seen in tissue water content, in acid-base balance, and in the concentrations of electrolytes, vitamin or mineral concentrations (6). These metabolic abnormalities may impair nutritional status and contribute to cancer cachexia via the depletion of fat, protein, water, and mineral stores (7).

Table 5.1   Metabolic Abnormalities Present in the Cancer State (5)

Carbohydrate Metabolism	Increased gluconeogenesis from amino acids and lactate
	Increased glucose disappearance and recycling
	Insulin resistance
Lipid Metabolism	Increased lypolysis
	Increased glycerol turnover
	Decreased lipogenesis
	Decreased lipoprotein lipase activity
	Free fatty acid hyperlipidemia
Protein Metabolism	Increased protein catabolism
	Increased whole body protein turnover
	Increased protein synthesis
	Decreased muscle protein synthesis

Cachexia and the Alteration to Normal Mechanisms of Metabolism

Cachexia is characterized by extreme weight loss, with depletion of both lean body muscle mass and adipose tissue, anorexia, early satiety, anemia, and emaciation (3). The normal physiologic conservation mechanisms seen during periods of acute starvation do not occur in the presence of a malignant tumor (8). Usually during periods of starvation, free fatty acids (FFA) from adipose tissue supply energy to the liver and muscle. The FFA are converted to ketone bodies (B-hydroxybutyrate and acetoacetate), which are then utilized by body tissues (Figure 5.1). Acting as a glucose substitute, ketone bodies signal the body to inhibit glucose utilization and induce protein and adipose tissue conservation mechanisms. Rates of gluconeogenesis and protein degradation from muscle mass decline along with insulin levels. Ketone bodies play an important role as an alternative energy source during periods of starvation.

Figure 5.1   Metabolic pathways of synthesis of the ketone bodies (D-B-hydroxybutyrate and acetoacetate) in the liver and their utilization in the brain and muscle (non-hepatic tissues). Ketones are transported from the liver to non-hepatic tissues via the circulation system. The terms NAD+, NADH, and COA refer to nicotinamide adenine dinucleotide, the reduced form of NAD+, and Coenzyme A, respectively.

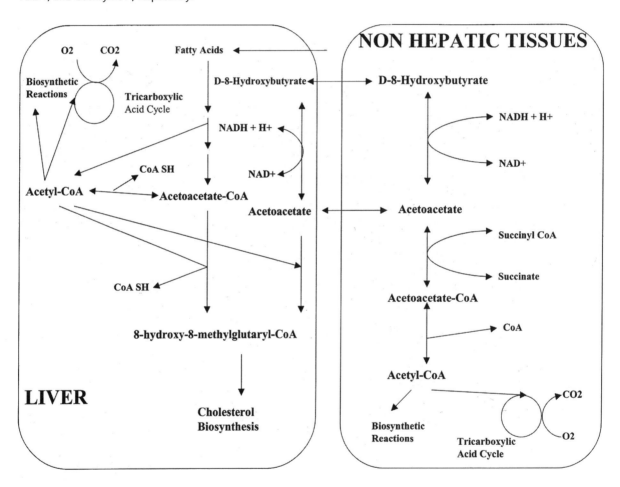

The Influence of Cytokines on Cachexia

These normal responses to starvation are not seen to the same degree in the presence of tumor malignancy. Inappropriately high energy consumption rates by the tumor could be contributing to the generalized wasting seen in cachectic cancer patients. There is documented evidence that increased rates of glucose turnover, body fat loss, and nonspecific inflammatory response mediated partly by proinflammatory cytokinens exist in the cachectic patient (8,9,10). There is a decrease in protein synthesis, with a decrease in circulating proteins, noted in some patients. High protein turnover and impaired muscle protein synthesis occur also (5).

Data indicate that certain cytokines, notably tumor necrosis factor (TNF-α) (11,12) and interleukin (IL)-1 and IL-6 and interferon-γ (13) may act as mediators of cachexia. Tumor necrosis factor is thought to inhibit the synthesis and activity of lipoprotein lipase (12). In clinical patients, TNF-α production may be increased, but there is inconsistent evidence to show that TNF-α is causally related to the metabolic changes observed in patients with cancer cachexia (4).

The Consequence of Altered Metabolism

The tumor's presence may alter the patient's ability and desire to eat. Side effects of traditional treatment modalities combine to further impair the nutritional status of the patient (5) (see Chapter 6, *Chemotherapy and Nutrition Implications;* Chapter 7, *Nutrition Concerns with the Radiation Therapy Patient;* Chapter 8, *Nutrition Implications of Surgical Oncology;* and Chapter 9, *Medical Nutrition Therapy in Bone Marrow Transplantation*). The overall impact of glucose intolerance, impaired insulin sensitivity, and increased caloric expenditure combined with reduced caloric intake due to anorexia, further exacerbate alterations in energy metabolism initiated by the tumor (8,14).

A significant increase in the rate of glucose turnover combined with increased energy demand by the tumor, contribute to increased energy expenditure and depletion of body fat stores observed in some cancer patients (15). Normal energy substrates that usually provide an alternate fuel supply during periods of stress or starvation are instead poorly metabolized by the tumor cells (16). Therefore, understanding the relationship between nutrient needs and tumor metabolism in the cancer patient is critical if nutritional intervention is to have a positive impact and improve the patient's outcome.

Change in Carbohydrate Metabolism

Cori Cycle Activity

A well-nourished adult in the basal or resting state will consume glucose at a rate of 140 g/day (560 kcal). Under typical metabolic conditions, oxidation of amino acids during normal tissue break down accounts for 75 g/day (375 kcal), and oxidation of triglycerides at 130 g/day (1170 kcal) accounts for the rest in a well-nourished adult. In the resting state approximately 20 g lactate are formed daily and are normally resynthesized back to glucose in an adult (17). This cyclic metabolic pathway, in which glucose is converted to lactic acid by glycolysis and then reconverted to glucose in the liver, is referred to as the Cori cycle (Figure 5.2). Abnormal elevation in Cori cycle activity has been noted in malnourished cancer patients and this increased activity is reported to account for up to 300 kcal/d loss of energy (18). The demand for glucose carbons by the tumor tissue can increase demand for glucose production by the liver, especially if glucose cannot be fully oxidized by the tumor tissue itself. This inability to effectively oxidize glucose may explain why some cancer patients exhibit an increase in Cori cycle activity and elevated glucose production (18).

Figure 5.2   Cori-type Cycling of Glucose and Lactate Between the Tumor and the Host

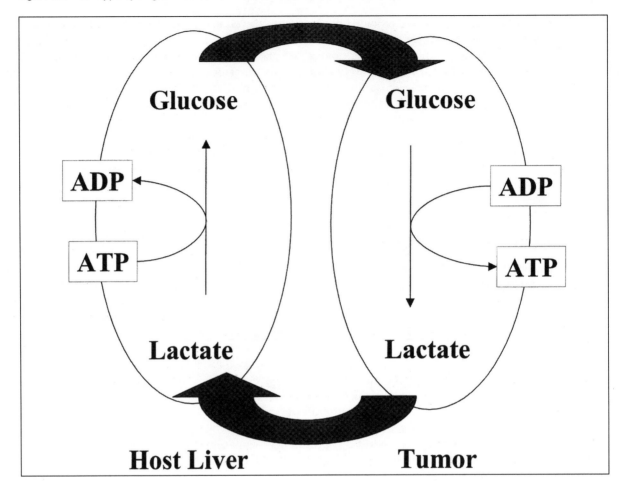

Increased Glycolysis and Lactate Production

Increased glucose uptake and lactate production have been measured in the forearm of cachectic cancer patients with esophageal cancer (19) and in various peripheral tissues (20). The increased lactate level and plasma lactate production rate in cancer patients is due to increased glycolysis and lactate release by the tumor tissue, and increased lactate release by skeletal muscle tissue. The precursors for glucose synthesis are provided by amino acids, primarily alanine, released from skeletal muscle tissue (21). Thus without appropriate antineoplastic treatment, the Cori cycle enables continual tumor growth in the wasted host (22).

Increased Gluconeogenesis

Increased rates of gluconeogenesis are critical in maintaining glucose homeostasis in the cancer patient (23). In order to meet the increased demands for glucose, the rates of glucose recycling and gluconeogenesis with alanine as primary precursor must be increased. Cachectic cancer patients have reduced plasma levels of alanine, glycine, and glutamine (19). Similarly, reduced levels of plasma alanine and other gluconeogenic precursors are also seen in diabetic patients. In the cancer patient, decreased plasma levels of these amino acids may be caused by an increase in their utilization by the liver for glucose production (19).

Increased Insulin Sensitivity

Although cancer patients are reported to have normal levels of circulating insulin and glucose, they may experience impaired insulin sensitivity (24). Glucose intolerance is documented by hyperglycemia and delayed clearance of blood glucose in some cancer patients after oral or intravenous glucose administration (2). Tumor induced hyperglycemia may result in a hyperinsulinemic state. In turn, the elevated insulin levels may stimulate DNA synthesis and cell proliferation in the epithelial component of the tumor. Elevated levels of free fatty acids which result from the hyperglycemic state could enhance further tumor growth (25). Further studies are needed to clarify the development of insulin resistance in cancer patients.

Changes in Lipid Metabolism
Lipid Mobilization and Hydrolysis

Alterations in lipid metabolism in cancer patients include alteration in body composition and increased lipid mobilization (Table 5.1). Studies indicate that hypermetabolic cancer patients have increased rates of lipolysis, fatty acid and glycerol turnover, and fatty acid oxidation (26, 27). Elevated plasma free fatty acids (FFA) and low respiratory quotients, as well as increased fat oxidation rates, suggest that the cancer patient has adapted to fatty acid metabolism on a whole-body level (28). This adaptive process can occur when the tumor mass is very small. It is associated with increased plasma lipid concentrations and changes in the plasma lipoprotein composition and plasma lipase activity. In addition to the increased mobilization, phospholipid biosynthesis may be affected during tumor growth. This effect may be the result of tumor produced lipolytic substances (27). Patients with malignancy that fail to suppress lipolysis after glucose administration will continue to oxidize fatty acids (29).

Changes in Protein Metabolism
Nitrogen Balance and Muscle Wasting

Protein functions as a critical reserve of metabolic fuel and may become seriously depleted during tumor growth. Various alterations in protein metabolism occur in cancer patients, including host nitrogen depletion, decreased muscle protein synthesis, increased protein catabolism in liver and skeletal muscle, and abnormal plasma amino acid levels (Table 5.1) (19,30). Negative nitrogen balance may be present in select patients with progressive malignancy (31). Consider that human tumors are rarely larger than 1% of body mass; changes in the patient's whole body protein metabolism is attributed to the degree of cachectic response via the type and stage of tumor present.

It has been noted both clinically and experimentally that tumor cells will use greater concentrations of circulating amino acid (32). Studies on the dynamics of protein metabolism in human subjects have shown that muscle tissue degradation in the whole body are elevated in patients with various types of cancer, a response similar to other conditions such as infection and injury (33).

Nutritional Implications
How Would Metabolic Changes Affect the Patient?

The presence of a malignant tumor may alter the body composition of the host. Specifically, the presence of a tumor may initiate a sequence of events which can lead to altered carbohydrate, lipid, and protein metabolism, and the potential depletion of the patient's body stores. Increased rates of anaerobic glycolysis by tumors will increase the consumption rates of glucose or gluconeogenic precursors during phases of active growth. These changes in host glucose and lactate metabolism may provide a biological advantage to the tumor (34). Insulin resistance and glucose intolerance in host tissue and increased gluconeogenesis may help maintain the circulating levels of these nutrients despite an increased demand by the host and tumor tissue (30) and a concomitant decrease in food intake triggered by anorexia (7).

Could Dietary Modulation Stimulate Tumor Growth?

Dietary modulation may be beneficial, yet the possibility exists that this might stimulate tumor growth (35). Efforts have been made to identify the ideal means to replete the host without simulating tumor growth (15, 36). The following effects have been reported in clinical studies.

- Supplementation of arginine may potentially stimulate the immune system, enhance wound healing, improve recovery time from trauma, and inhibit tumor growth rates (33,37).
- Supplementation of ketones as the primary energy source may reduce the fall in urinary nitrogen levels and initiate protein conservation in the host (15).

A number of tumors specifically metabolize glucose so the administration of a concentrated lipid source of energy (ie, medium chain triglyceride oil) may reduce the glucose substrate available to the tumor (38). Supplying adequate caloric substrates to the host in a form which can not be utilized by the tumor may inhibit tumor growth by decreasing catabolism of host body stores (15,34,39). Data suggests that dietary modulations may be used to improve the patient's nutritional status and prevent exacerbation of cachexia; however, further research is needed. Any potential tumor growth enhancement could be used to the clinician's advantage. By stimulation of the cells' proliferative phase, specific chemotherapeutic agents might be targeted more effectively. Thus, understanding the biochemical relationships between tumor-host interactions are necessary if nutritional intervention is to offer therapeutic benefits.

Summary

The presence of a tumor has been shown to affect the patient's biochemical and metabolic functions, which impact upon normal metabolism. Changes in energy expenditure, baseline metabolism, and enzyme activity occur. The result is an alteration in carbohydrate, lipid, and protein metabolism and in energy requirements. Understanding the relationship between nutritional needs and the effects of tumor metabolism is essential if prescribed nutritional intervention is to improve a patient's status. Given these concerns, the following chapters provide further details on appropriate nutrition intervention strategies which target the special needs of the cancer patient.

References

1. Tisdale MJ. Biology of Cachexia. *J Natl Cancer Inst*. 1997;89:1763-1773.
2. Heber D, Chelbowski RT, Ishibash DE, Herrold JN, Block JB. Abnormalities in glucose and protein metabolism in non-cachectic lung cancer patients. *Cancer Res* 1982;42:4815-4819.
3. Sauer LA, Dauchy RT. Pathways of Energy Metabolism in Cancer. In: Watson RR, Mufti SI, eds. *Nutrition and Cancer Prevention*. Boca Raton, Fla: CRC Press; 1996;119-137.
4. Keller U. Pathophysiology of cancer cachexia. *Supportive Care Cancer* 1993; 1:290-294.
5. Laviano A, Meguid MM. Nutritional issues in cancer management. *Nutrition* 1996;12(5):358-371.
6. Buzby GP, Mullen JL, Stein TP, Miller EE, Hobbs CL, Rosato EF. Host-tumor interaction and nutrient supply. *Cancer* 1980;45:2924-2948.
7. Bass FB, Cox RH. The need for dietary counseling of cancer patients as indicated by nutrient and supplement intake. *J Am Diet Assoc* 1995;95(11): 1319-1321.
8. Tayek JA. A review of cancer cachexia and abnormal glucose metabolism in humans with cancer. *J Am Coll Nutr* 1992;11(4):445-456.

9. Emery PW, Carpenter TTA, Obeid OA. Alterations in postprandial glycogen and lipid synthesis in cachectic tumor-bearing rats. *Nutr Cancer* 1993;20:231-240.

10. Espat NJ, Moldawer LL, Copeland EM. Cytokine-mediated alterations in host metabolism prevent nutritional repletion in cachectic cancer patients. *J Surg Oncol* 1995;58:77-82.

11. Yoneda T, Alsina MA, Chavez JB, Bonewald L, Nishimura R, Mundy GR. Evidence that tumor necrosis factor plays a pathogenetic role in the paraneoplastic syndrome of cachexia, hypercalcemia, and leukocytosis in a human tumor in nude mice. *J Clin Invest* 1991;87:977-985.

12. Stovroff MC, Fracker DL, Norton JA. Cachectin activity in the serum of cachectic, tumor-bearing rats. *Arch Surg* 1989;124:94-99.

13. Jablons DM, McIntosh JK, Mule JJ. Induction of interferon-b2 /interlukin-6 (IL-6) by cytokine administration and detection of circulating IL-6 in the tumor bearing state. *Ann NY Acad Sci.* 1989;577:157-166.

14. Tayek J.A. Reduced non-oxidative glucose utilization in cancer patients is associated with a low tri-iodothyronine concentration. *J Am Coll Nutr* 1995; 14(4):341-348.

15. Rothkopf M. Fuel utilization in neoplastic disease: implications for the use of nutritional support in cancer patients. *Nutrition* 1990;6:14s-16s.

16. Rofe AM, Bias R, Conyers RAJ. Ketone body metabolism in tumor bearing rats. *Biochem. J* 1986;233:485-491.

17. Dills W.L. Nutritional and physiological consequences of tumor glycolysis. *Parasitology* 1993;107:S177-S186.

18. Eden D, Edstrom S, Bennegard K, Schersten T, Lundholm K. Glucose flux in relation to energy expenditure with and without cancer during periods of fasting and feeding. *Cancer Res* 1984;44:1718-1724.

19. Burt ME, Aoki TT, Gorschboth CM, Brennan MF. Peripheral tissue metabolism in cancer bearing man. *Ann Surg* 1983;198:685-691.

20. Albert JD, Legaspi A, Horowitz GD, Tracey KFJ, Brennan MF, Lowry SF. Peripheral tissue metabolism in man with varied disease states and similar weight loss. *J Surg Res* 1986;40:374-381.

21. Luque P, Paredes S, Segura JA, Nunez de Castro I, Medina MA. Mutual effect of glucose and glutamine on their utilization by tumor cells. *Biochem Int* 1990; 21:9-15.

22. Cori CF, Cori GT. The Carbohydrate Metabolism of Tumors. *J Biol Chem* 1925;65:397-405.

23. Kallinowski F, Vaupel P, Runkel S, Berg G, Fortmeyer HP, Baessler KH, Wagner K, Mueller-Klieser W, Walenta S. Glucose uptake, lactate release, ketone body turnover, metabolic micromilieu, and pH distributions in human breast cancer xenografts in nude rats. *Cancer Res* 1988;48:7264-7272.

24. Yam D. Insulin-cancer relationships: possible dietary implication. *Medical Hypothesis* 1992;38:111-117.

25. Iguchi I, Takasugi N, Nishimura N, Kusunoki S. Correlation between mammary tumor and blood glucose, serum insulin, and free fatty acids in mice. *Cancer Res* 1989;49:821-825.

26. Beck SA, Groundwater P, Barton C, Tisdale MJ. Alterations in serum lipolytic activity of cancer patients with response to therapy. *Br J Cancer* 1990;62:822-825.

27. Groundwater P, Beck SA, Barton C, Adamson C, Ferrier IN, Tisdale MJ. Alteration of serum and urinary lipolytic activity with weight loss in cachexic cancer patients. *Br J Cancer* 1990;62:816-821.

28. Klein S, Wolfe RA Whole body lipolysis and triglyceride fatty acid cycling in cachectic cancer patients with esophageal cancer. *J Clin Invest.* 1990;86:1403-1408.

29. Legaspi A, Jeevanadam M, Starnes HF, Brennan MF. Whole body lipid and energy metabolism in the cancer patient. *Metabolism* 1987; 36(10):958-963.

30. Minn H, Nuutila P, Lindholm P, Ruotsalainen U, Bergman J, Teras M, Knuuti MJ. In vivo effects of insulin on tumor and skeletal muscle glucose metabolism in patients with lymphoma. *Cancer* 1994;73:1490-1498.

31. Pisters PW, Brennan, MF. Amino acid metabolism in human cancer cachexia. *Ann Rev Nutr* 1990;10:107-132.

32. Norton JA, Burt ME, Brennan MF. In vivo utilization of substrate by human sarcoma-bearing limbs. *Cancer* 1980;45:2934-2939.

33. Garlick PJ, McNurlan MA. Protein metabolism in cancer patients. *Biochimie* 1994;76:713-717.

34. Daly JM, Shinkwin M. Nutrition and the Cancer Patient. In: Murphy GP, Lawrence W, Lenhard RE, eds. *American Cancer Society Textbook of Clinical Oncology.* 2nd edition, Atlanta, Ga: American Cancer Society, Inc; 1995;580–596.

35. Langen KJ, Braun U, Kops ER, Kuwert T, Nebeling B, Feinendegen LE. The influence of plasma glucose levels on fluorine-18-fluordeoxygluoxe uptake in bronchial carcinomas. *J Nucl Med* 1993;34:355–359.

36. Franchi F, Rossi-Fanelli F, Seminara P, Cascino A, Barone C, Scucchi L. Cell kinetics of gastrointestinal tumors after different nutritional regiments. *J Clin Gastroenterol* 1991;13(3):313–315.

37. Heys S.D, Gough DB, Khan L, Eremin O. Nutritional pharmacology and malignant disease: a therapeutic modality in patients with cancer. *Br J Surg* 1996;83:608–619.

38. Nebeling L, Miraldi F, Shurin S, Lerner E. Effects of Ketogenic Diet on Tumor Metabolism and Nutritional Status in Pediatric Oncology Patients: Two Case Reports. *J Am Coll Nutr* 1995;14:202–208.

39. Nebeling L, Lerner E. Implementing a ketogenic diet in pediatric oncology patients. *J Am Diet Assoc* 1995;95:693–697.

6

Chemotherapy and Nutrition Implications

Barbara Eldridge, RD

Chemotherapy is the use of chemical agents or medications to treat cancer. Whereas surgery and radiation therapy are used to treat localized tumors, chemotherapy is a systemic therapy which affects the whole body. (1) The actions of antineoplastic chemotherapeutic agents can be cytotoxic to normal cells as well as malignant cells, in particular those cells with a rapid turnover such as bone marrow, hair follicles, and oral and intestinal mucosa.

Oncology patients may experience altered food intake from chemotherapy-induced side effects which can include nausea, vomiting, anorexia, mucositis, esophagitis, fatigue, and alterations in bowel habits (constipation, bloating or diarrhea). Normal gut function may also be affected because of damage to the cells that line the gastrointestinal tract. Resulting changes in digestion and absorption can further compromise nutrition status. These agents can also adversely impact hepatic and renal function. Chemotherapy-induced bone marrow suppression can cause anemia, neutropenia, and thrombocytopenia. The severity of experienced side effects relates to single- or combination-agent therapy, dose administration (ie high-dose or dose intensification), planned number of cycles, individual response, medications, and current health status.

Several factors need to be considered when evaluating a patient's response to chemotherapy. Important factors include how much tumor burden is present, use of combined treatment modalities (surgery, radiation therapy and/or chemotherapy), existing medical conditions, nutrition status, and the goal or intent of the planned therapy.

The goals of antineoplastic treatment are:
- Cure   - to obtain a complete response to treatment of a specific cancer
- Control   - to extend the length of life when cure is not possible
  - to obscure microscopic metastases after tumors are surgically removed
  - to shrink tumors before surgery or radiation therapy
- Palliation - to provide comfort when cure or control is not possible
  - to improve quality of life
  - to reduce tumor burden, therefore helping to relieve cancer-related symptoms such as pain and organ obstruction (1,2).

Table 6.1 describes the effects of chemotherapeutic agents and their mechanisms of action.

Table 6.1 Classification of Antineoplastic Chemotherapeutic Agents

Drug	Mechanism of Action
Alkylating Agents	Cell-cycle, phase-nonspecific agents that substitute an alkyl group for a hydrogen atom; results in cross-linking of DNA strands and interference with replication of DNA and transcription of RNA
Antibiotics	Inhibit cell division by binding to DNA; interferes with RNA transcription
Antimetabolites	Interferes with nucleic acid synthesis by substituting drug for purines or pyrimidines necessary for normal cellular function
Hormones	Alter cellular metabolism by changing body hormonal milieu for unfavorable tumor growth
Miscellaneous	
Platinum coordination complexes	Cross-link DNA strands that inhibit DNA synthesis
Substituted ureas	Cell-cycle specific agents that inhibit DNA synthesis and ribonucleotide reductases
Methylhydrazine derivatives	Cause breakage of the chromosome with separation of DNA strands
Plant Alkaloids	Inhibit mitotic spindle formation and block mitosis
Biological Response Modifiers	Modify host biologic responses to tumor

Source: *BMT/PBSCT Nutrition Care Criteria Manual*, Drug/Nutrient Interaction Table 1. Clinical Nutrition, Fred Hutchinson Cancer Research Center, Seattle, Wash:1995.

Supportive Therapies

The use of supportive therapies may help to reduce chemotherapy morbidity and mortality. Aggressive and thorough management of nutrition-related side effects throughout the patient's treatment course can have a positive effect on nutrition status and well being (5). Refer to Appendix A for nutrition recommendations for managing treatment-related side effects and Chapter 4, *Calorie, Protein, Fluid, and Micronutrient Requirements of the Oncology Patient,* for determining estimated energy, protein, and fluid requirements. Other supportive therapies include the use of blood products to manage episodes of treatment-induced bone marrow suppression, use of prophylactic antibiotics to minimize the occurrence and severity of treatment-related infections of the urinary and gastrointestinal tracts, and medications such as antidiarrheals and antiemetics to aid in the management of chemotherapy induced diarrhea and nausea. (See Appendix B, *Common Supportive Drug Therapies Used with Oncology Patients.*)

Classification of Antineoplastic Chemotherapeutic Agents

The three main classifications of antineoplastic chemotherapeutic agents are cytotoxics, hormonals, and immunologicals. These agents are effective because they interfere with cellular metabolism and replication, which results in cell death. Chemotherapeutic agents vary in their modes of action and they are classified as cell cycle-(phase) specific, or cell cycle-(phase) nonspecific. Cell cycle-specific agents have their effect during a specific phase or phases of the cell cycle. Cell cycle-nonspecific agents act on cells whether they are actively dividing in any phase of the cell cycle or in the resting (non-replicating) state. (3)

The five phases of the cell cycle are:
1. Resting Phase—Gap 0 (G0): Cells are not committed to cell division
2. Post Mitotic Phase—Gap 1 (G1): RNA and protein synthesis
3. Synthesis—(S): DNA synthesis
4. Premitotic or Postsynthetic Phase—Gap 2 (G2): RNA and protein synthesis
5. Mitosis—(M): Cellular division occurs (3,5,8)

Cytotoxics include alkylating agents, antibiotics, antimetabolites, miscellaneous agents, and plant alkaloids. These agents have specific mechanisms of action and are toxic to malignant cells and normal host cells that have a high replication rate. Hormonals are used in the treatment of hormone sensitive cancers such as prostate, endometrial, and breast cancer. (5) Hormone therapy can alter the body's hormonal environment, causing changes in the cancer cell's normal growth, and the suppression or removal of the stimulus for tumor growth. Examples of immunologicals include Interluken-2, which is FDA approved for the treatment of metastatic renal cell cancer and for use in many ongoing clinical trials, and granulocyte colony stimulating factor (G-CSF) which is used to treat febrile neutropenia following bone marrow suppressing chemotherapy.

Nutritional Implications of Chemotherapeutic Agents

Information about cytotoxics, hormonals, and immunologicals and their nutritional implications are outlined in Table 6.2. To apply the information:
- Identify the chemotherapeutic agent(s) being used.
- Locate each chemotherapeutic agent on the table.
- Determine which treatment related side effects are anticipated.
- Formulate a nutrition care plan which would include discussion of potential treatment related side effects; their nutrition implications and management suggestions.

Example

Diagnosis: A 40-year-old premenopausal woman with poorly differentiated, infiltrating ductal carcinoma of the breast and positive lymph nodes

Treatment Plan: (Adjuvant Therapy)
- Surgery - Modified Radical Mastectomy
- Radiation Therapy to the breast and surrounding tissue
- Chemotherapy - 6 cycles of CMF
  - Cyclophosphamide (Cytoxan-tm)
  - Methotrexate
  - 5 Fluorouracil (5 FU)

Anticipated Side Effects May Include:
- Myleosuppression   moderate to severe
- Nausea/Vomiting   moderate to severe
- Fatigue   yes
- Anorexia   yes
- Mucositis/Esophagitis   yes
- Diarrhea   yes
- Renal   yes
- Hepatic   yes

Nutrition Care Plan Management Suggestions:
- Safe food handling (neutropenic precautions)
- Nausea and vomiting management suggestions
- Tips for improving appetite, maintaining weight, and incorporating nutritionally dense foods into daily eating plan
- Tips for managing treatment related fatigue—such as use of easy-to-prepare foods and seeking assistance from friends and family in meal planning and preparation
- Use of a soft-textured, bland diet to aid in management of sore/tender mouth and throat
- Use of a low fiber diet to aid in diarrhea management
- Encourage the intake of fluids for adequate hydration.
- Encourage the avoidance of high fat, greasy or fried foods.
- Encourage open communication with the healthcare team with regard to any nutrition problems encountered and efficacy of management suggestions.

Table 6.2 Nutritional Implications of Chemotherapeutics Agents (4,6-9)

Antineoplastic Agent	Myelo-suppression	Nausea & Vomiting	Anorexia	Mucositis & Esophagitis	Diarrhea	Renal	Hepatic	Other
CYTOTOXICS								
bleomycin Blenoxane® (Bristol Myers Oncology, Princeton, NJ)	None to mild	Mild to moderate	x	x				Weight loss; xerostomia; pulmonary fibrosis
busulfan Myleran® (GlaxoWellcome, Research Triangle Park, NC) Buslfex® (Orphan Medical, Minnetonka, Minn)	Mild to moderate	Mild	x				x	May cause weight loss; pulmonary fibrosis
carboplatin Paraplatin® (Bristol Myers Oncology, Princeton, NJ)	Moderate	Moderate			x	x		Ototoxicity
carmustine BCNU® (Bristol Myers Oncology, Princeton, NJ)	Moderate to severe	Mild to moderate	x	x		x	x	Pulmonary toxicity; phlebitis
chlorambucil Leukeran® (GlaxoWellcome, Research Triangle Park, NC)	Mild to moderate	Mild						Pulmonary fibrosis
cisplatin CDDP Platinol® (Bristol Myers Oncology, Princeton, NJ)	Mild to moderate	Severe	x		x	x		Decreased serum Mg, K, Zn; renal tubular necrosis; metallic taste; ototoxicity
cyclophosphamide Cytoxan® (Mead Johnson Oncology, Princeton, NJ)		Moderate to severe	x	x		x		Xerostomia; abdominal pain; pulmonary fibrosis
cytarabine ARA-C	Moderate to severe	Severe	x	x	x	x	x	Flu-like symtoms
dacarbazine DTIC DTIC-Dome® (Bayer Corporation, West Haven, Conn)	Moderate	Severe		x	x			Metallic taste; flu-like symptoms
dactinomycin Actinomycin-D, ACT	Moderate to severe	Moderate to severe		x-severe*	x			Xerostomia; taste alterations; radiation recall
daunorubicin citrate Daunomycin® (Wyeth-Ayerst Laboratories, Philadelphia, Pa)	Moderate to severe	Moderate	x	x-severe*	x			Xerostomia; change in taste acuity; cardiotoxicity
daunorubicin liposomal Daunoxome® (Nexstar Pharmaceuticals, Boulder, Colo)	x	x			x			Fatigue; headache; cough; dyspnea

continued

Antineoplastic Agent	Myelo-suppression	Nausea & Vomiting	Anorexia	Mucositis & Esophagitis	Diarrhea	Renal	Hepatic	Other
docetaxel Taxotere® (Rhone-Poulene Rorer Pharm., Collegeville, Pa)	Severe	Mild					x	
doxorubicin Adriamycin® (Pharmacia & Upjohn, Kalamazoo, Mich)	Moderate to severe	Moderate	x	x-severe*	x			Xerostomia; cardiotoxicity; radiation recall
epirubicin HCl Ellence® (Pharmacia & Upjohn, Peapack, NJ)		x			x			Hair loss; stomatitis; cardiotoxicity
etoposide VP-16-23	Moderate	Mild to moderate	x	x	x		x	Hypotension; fever
floxuridine FUDR® (Roche Laboratories, Nutley, NJ)	Mild to moderate	Mild	x	x	x	x	x	Blurred vision; lethargy; vertigo
5-Fluorouracil 5-FU, 5-Fluorouracil	Moderate	Moderate		x-severe*	x		x	Taste alterations; avoid pyridoxine supplements; cardiotoxicity
gemcitabine Gemzar® (Eli Lilly and Company, Indianapolis, Ind)	Mild to moderate	Moderate		x	x	x		Fever; rash; dyspnea
hydroxyurea Hydrea® (Burlex Laboratories, Wayne, NJ)	Moderate	Mild to moderate	x	x	x			
irenotecan Camptosar® (Pharmacia & Upjohn, Kalamazoo, Mich)	Moderate	Moderate to severe	x		x-severe*			Fever; abdominal pain; asthenia
ifosfamide Ifex® (Mead Johnson Oncology, Princeton, NJ)	Mild to moderate					x		Confusion; lethargy
L-asparaginase Elspar® (Merck & Co, West Point, Pa)		Moderate	x	x		x	x	Decreased protein synthesis; hypoalbuminemia; pancreatitis; weight loss; hyperglycemia
lomustine CCNU CeeNu® (Bristol Myers Oncology, Princeton, NJ)	Severe	Mild to moderate	x	x		x	x	Pulmonary fibrosis
mechlorethamine Nitrogen Mustard, HN2 Mustargen® (Merck &Co, West Point, Pa)	Moderate	Severe	x		x			Metallic taste; fever; chills; tinnitis

continued

Antineoplastic Agent	Myelo-suppression	Nausea & Vomiting	Anorexia	Mucositis & Esophagitis	Diarrhea	Renal	Hepatic	Other
melphalan Alkeran® (GlaxoWellcome, Research Triangle Park, NC)	Moderate	Mild to moderate						Pulmonary fibrosis
mercaptopurine Purinethol® (GlaxoWellcome, Research Triangle Park, NC)	Moderate	Mild to moderate	x	x	x	x	x	Biliary stasis; cholestatic jaundice; pancreatis
methotrexate MTX	Moderate	Mild to moderate	x	x-severe*	x	x	x	Decreased absorption of B12, fat and D-xylose; change in taste acuity; pneumonitis
mitomycin Mitomycin-C, MTC Mutamycin® (Bristol Myers Oncology, Princeton, NJ)	Severe	Moderate	x	x	x	x	x	Hypercalcemia
mitoxantrone Novantrone® (Immunex, Seattle, Wash)	Mild to moderate	Mild		x	x		x	
plicamycin Mithracin® (Miles, West Haven, Conn)	Mild to moderate	Moderate to severe	x	x-severe*	x	x	x	Decreased Serum Ca, PO4; fever; coagulopathy
paclitaxel Taxol® (Bristol Myers Squibb, Princeton, NJ)	Severe	Mild		x			x	Fatigue
procarbazine Matulane® (Roche Laboratories Nutley, NJ)	Moderate to severe	Moderate to severe	x	x	x	x	x	Monoamine oxidase inhibitor; low tyramine diet; decreased serum K, Ca, PO4
streptozocin Zanosar® (Pharmacia & Upjohn, Kalamazoo, Mich)	Mild	Severe	x		x	x	x	Hypoglycemia
thioguanine 6-Thioguanine, TG Thioguanine® (GlaxoWellcome, Research Triangle Park, NC)	Severe	Mild	x	x	x	x	x	
topotecan Hycamtin® (SmithKline Beecham, Philadelphia, Pa)	Severe	Moderate to severe	x		x			Fever
vinblastine sulfate Velban® (Eli Lilly & Company, Indianapolis, Ind)	Severe	Mild to moderate		x	x		x	Constipation

continued

Antineoplastic Agent	Myelo-suppression	Nausea & Vomiting	Anorexia	Mucositis & Esophagitis	Diarrhea	Renal	Hepatic	Other
vincristine sulfate Oncovin® (*Eli Lilly & Company, Indianapolis, Ind*)	Mild	Mild	x	x	x		x	Peripheral neuropathy; abdominal pain; hyponatremia; alternating diarrhea and constipation
vinorelbine tartate Navelbine® (*GlaxoWellcome Research Triangle Park, NC*)	Moderate to severe	Moderate	x		x			Constipation
HORMONALS								
Glucocorticoids: **prednisone, dexamethasone,** Decadron® (*Merck & Company, West Point, Pa*)		Mild						Hyperphagia; sodium and fluid retention; GI upset; glucose intolerance; potassium wasting; hyperlipidemia; osteoporosis; negative nitrogen balance
Androgens: **fluoxymesterone**		Mild						Fluid retention; hypercalcemia; increased growth velocity
Antiandrogens: **flutamide** Eulexin® (*Nexstar Pharm, Inc., Boulder, Colo*)		x			x	x		Hot flashes; decreased libido; impotence
Antiestrogens: **tamoxifen citrate** Novaldex® (*Zeneca Pharmaceuticals, Wilmington, Del*)	Mild	Mild	x					Bone pain; edema fluid retention; hypercalcemia; hot flashes
Estrogens: **diethylstilbesterol** DES		Mild	x					Fluid and sodium retention; hypertension; hypercalcemia
Progestins: **megestrol acetate** Megace® (*Mead Johnson Oncology, Princeton, NJ*) Depo-Provera® (*Pharmacia & Upjohn, Kalamazoo, Mich*)		Mild						Increased appetite; fluid retention; weight gain; hypercalcemia
Gonadotropin-Releasing Hormone Analog: **leuprolide** Lupron® (*TAP Pharm, Deerfield, Ill*)		Mild						Bone pain

continued

Antineoplastic Agent	Myelo-suppression	Nausea & Vomiting	Anorexia	Mucositis & Esophagitis	Diarrhea	Renal	Hepatic	Other
IMMUNOLOGICALS								
Hematopeitic Agents **epoetin alfa** Erythropoietin, EPO Procrit® *(OrthoBiotech, Raritan, NJ)* Epogen® *(Amgen, Thousand Oaks, Calif)*								Fever; decreased transferrin and ferritin levels; iron supplementation may be necessary
filgastim Granulocyte Colony Stimulating Factor, GM-CSF Neupogen® *(Amgen, Thousand Oaks, Calif)*	Mild to moderate	x	x	x	x			Bone pain; flu-like symptoms; fever
sargramostin Granulocyte Macrophage Colony Stimulating Factor, GM-CSF Leukine® *(Immunex, Seattle, Wash)*	Mild to moderate	x						Bone pain; flu-like symptoms; fever
IMMUNOLOGICALS								
rituximab Rituxan® *(IDEC/Genetech, San Diego, Calif)*	x	x						Fever; chills; rash
trastuzumab Herceptin® *(Genetech, San Francisco, Calif)*	x	Mild				x		Fever; chills; rash
interferon alfa Alfa n-I Lymphoblastiod Wellferon® *(GlaxoWellcome, Research Triangle Park, NC)*	Mild to moderate	Mild to moderate	x					Weight loss or weight gain; flu-like symptoms
aldesleukin Interleukin-2, IL-2 Proleukin® *(Chiron Therapeutics, Emeryville, Calif)*	Moderate	Moderate						Weight loss or weight gain; hypotension; chills; fatigue; capillary leak syndrome

*Dose Dependent

Reprinted with permission from *Drug/Nutrient Interaction BMT/PBSCT Nutrition Care Criteria.* Seattle, Wash: Clinical Nutrition, Fred Hutchinson Cancer Research Center;1995.

References

1. Dollinger M, Rosenbaum EH. What Happens in Chemotherapy. In: *Everyone's Guide to Chemotherapy*. 2nd ed. Kansas City, Mo: Sommerville House Books Ltd;1994.

2. Powell LL, Fishman MA, Mrozek-Orlowski, M. *Principles of Cancer Chemotherapy. Guidelines and Recommendations for Practice*. Pittsburgh, Pa: Oncology Nursing Press, Inc;1996.

3. Tenebaum L. The Cell Cycle Chemotherapy. In: *Cancer Chemotherapy: A Reference Guide*. Philadelphia, Pa: WB Saunders;1989.

4. Research dietitians and clinical nutrition specialists of the Fred Hutchinson Cancer Research Center, Swedish Medical Center, and Veterans Administration Medical Center. Drug-Nutrient Tables. In: *BMT/PBSCT Nutrition Care Criteria*. Seattle, Wash: Clinical Nutrition, Fred Hutchinson Cancer Research Center;1995.

5. Holleb AI, Fink DJ, Murphy GP. *American Cancer Society Textbook of Clinical Oncology*. Atlanta, Ga: American Cancer Society, Inc;1991.

6. Fischer DS, Knobf MT, Durlage HJ. *The Cancer Chemotherapy Handbook*. 4th ed. St. Louis, Mo.: Mosby Yearbook, Inc;1993.

7. Koeller J, Fields S. Toxic Reactions of Most Commonly Used Antineoplastics - Chemotherapy Reference Card. [Currently part of Pharmacia/Upjohn Inc, Peapack, NJ.] Adria Laboratories;1990.

8. Baird SB, McCorkle R, Grant M. Medical Oncology: The Agents. In: *Cancer Nursing A Comprehensive Textbook*. Philadelphia, Pa: WB Saunders;1991.

9. *Facts and Comparisons 2000*. St. Louis, Mo: Wolter Kluwer Company;2000.

7

Nutrition Concerns with the Radiation Therapy Patient

Christine Gail Polisena MS, MBA, RD

Radiation therapy poses risks for developing nutrition problems which can result in significant weight loss. An understanding of the action of radiation therapy and its nutrition-related side effects will assist the dietetics professional in the development and management of nutrition care for this population. Appropriate nutrition screening and medical nutrition therapy can decrease the impact of side effects, help with weight maintenance, shorten recovery period after treatment, and improve quality of life.

What is Radiation Therapy?

Radiation therapy may be employed in the cure or palliation of treatment of solid tumors. Radiation therapy (i.e. total body irradiation [TBI]) is also used in the management and treatment of hematological cancers (leukemia, lymphoma). Radiation therapy damages the DNA of cells so the cells cannot continue to divide and grow. All cells in the treatment field are affected by radiation, but normal healthy cells recover more quickly than cancer cells. Tolerance of normal tissue to radiation therapy is the limiting factor for total dose administered. Therefore, radiation therapy is delivered in multiple fractions to allow recovery of normal tissue from sublethal damage and to maximize total dosage that may be administered to the tumor.

There are three types of radiation therapy treatments:

- **External beam** Radiation is directed at patient externally from a linear accelerator or cobalt unit, frequently causing nutrition-related side effects.
- **Brachytherapy** Radioactive material is placed directly into or next to the tumor to deliver a highly localized dose, in cervical or lung cancer for example. Nutrition-related side effects do not usually occur.
- **Stereotaxis** Radiation is aimed and delivered by a well-defined narrow beam to extremely hard-to-reach places, using a high dose per fraction. Brain tumors and arteriovenous malformations are examples of sites where stereotaxis radiation is used. Nutrition-related side effects do not usually occur.

The most common radiation treatment form, external beam radiation, is discussed further in this chapter.

The radiation oncologist determines the type of radiation treatment, area to irradiate, total dose, and number of fractions or treatments. Before treatment begins, a simulation reproducing the patient's planned treatment takes place. The tumor area is localized and lead blocks (to shield normal tissue) or immobilization devices are produced. The radiation field is marked on the patient's skin with a permanent marker or tattoos.

Radiation therapy is usually given 5 days a week for a period lasting from 2 to 7 weeks. Although most patients are treated once a day, some patients may receive treatments twice daily. A patient may receive treatment to one or more fields. The treatment takes 15 to 20 minutes each day with the patient feeling no pain or sensation during delivery of the radiation (1).

Nutrition-Related Side Effects

There are a number of side effects that are common among persons receiving radiation therapy. Radiation to the head and neck area often causes problems with taste, thick saliva, dry mouth, and dysphagia. Radiation to the abdomen and pelvis may cause problems with diarrhea, malabsorption, gas, and nausea. Table 7.1 lists the nutrition-related side effects of radiation therapy, based on cancer type or site. See further information regarding the management of nutrition-related problems secondary to cancer in Appendix A.

The side effects of radiation therapy depend on the area irradiated, total dose, fractionation, duration, and volume irradiated. Side effects can be acute (occur during treatment) or chronic (continue to or occur after treatment is over). Acute side effects begin around the second or third week of treatment. They peak about two-thirds of the way through treatment and last 2 to 3 weeks after treatment is completed. Taste and saliva changes due to head and neck radiation can take months to improve and may never return to baseline. Irradiation to the pelvic area where bowel is in the treatment field may cause lasting radiation enteritis.

Radiation therapy patients develop many of the nutrition-related side effects of treatment detailed in Table 7.1.

Table 7.1   Nutrition-Related Side Effects of Radiation Therapy (2,3)

Type of Cancer/Area Radiated	Acute Side Effects	Chronic Side Effects
Central nervous system (brain, spinal column)	Nausea Vomiting	
Head and neck areas (tongue, larynx, pharynx, tonsils, nasopharynx, salivary gland)	Mucositis Sore mouth and throat Dysphagia Odynophagia Xerostomia Loss of taste Dysgeusia Alteration or loss of smell Dysomia	Xerostomia Loss of taste Dental caries Ulcers Osteoradionecrosis Trismus
Thorax areas (lung, esophagus, breast)	Dysphagia Heartburn	Fibrosis Stenosis Perforations Fistula
Abdominal and pelvic areas (cervical, prostate, pancreatic, uterine, colon, rectal)	Anorexia Nausea Vomiting Diarrhea Gas and bloating Acute colitis and enteritis Choleretic enteropathy	Diarrhea Maldigestion Malabsorption Chronic colitis and enteritis Ulcer Stricture Obstruction Perforation Fistula

A random sampling of 50 patients in a radiation therapy department revealed that 41% of patients had experienced weight loss, 76% of patients experienced at least one nutrition related problem, 36% of patients ate less food than before their illness, and 20% took liquid nutritional supplements. Seventy-two percent of the patients responded that they would use the services of a dietitian if available (4). This indicates a need for nutrition-screening and counseling intervention in radiation therapy patients.

Studies looking at the prognosis of radiation therapy patients and nutrition assessment have found that skin anergy can be a predictor of survival (5,6). Yet it has been difficult to demonstrate improved survival or tumor control due to improved nutrition status, weight maintenance, or nutrition intervention (7,8). Patients do, however, perceive a benefit from nutrition therapy in terms of symptom relief and improvement in weight, as well as finding educational material and nutrition supplement samples helpful (9).

Nutrition Screening and Referral of Radiation Therapy Patients

Patients undergoing radiation therapy are at risk of developing nutrition problems. Therefore, screening of this population is important and should be the responsibility of all members of the healthcare team. The following are guidelines for screening and referral of patients receiving radiation therapy.

Screening

All radiation therapy patients should be screened for nutrition risk at simulation or during the first week of treatment, and weekly thereafter.

Patients can be screened by a dietetics professional (i.e. dietetic technician, registered dietitian), nurse, radiation therapist, physicians assistant, or physician. Need for nutrition intervention may be determined by use of a screening tool such as:
• Patient Generated-Subjective Global Assessment (PG-SGA) (see Chapter 2)
• weight loss guidelines: greater than or equal to 5-pound weight loss in one month, greater than or equal to 2 pound weight loss in one week, 1% to 2% weight loss in a week, or 5% weight loss in a month (10)
• patient concern about his or her nutrition status
• alternative diet program, such as macrobiotic
• excessive intake of vitamin and mineral supplements
• patient appears malnourished with muscle wasting or subcutaneous fat losses
• patient is undergoing adjuvant chemotherapy
• by diagnosis

The cancers that are most likely to have nutrition-related side effects are those involving the head and neck, lung, esophagus, prostate, cervix, uterus, colon, rectum, and pancreas. Head and neck cancer patients are at greatest risk of developing significant nutrition problems and severe weight loss. This population may present to radiation therapy with pre-existing malnutrition (11). The larger the field of irradiation and/or inclusion of the oral cavity/oropharynx, the greater the percentage of weight loss (12). Brown studied patients with lung cancer undergoing radiation and found that the elderly, males, and patients who continued to smoke have increased risk of experiencing cancer-related weight loss (13).

Referral to a Dietetics Professional

If a patient is at risk of developing nutrition-related side effects from treatment or is malnourished at simulation, the patient should be seen by a dietetics professional within the first week of treatment. The goal is to provide patients with information to help them manage potential nutrition side effects before they occur, rather than waiting until problems develop and/or weight loss occurs.

- Patients should be weighed and monitored for nutrition-related side effects weekly. Certain diagnoses such as head and neck, pancreas, or esophageal cancer may require daily weighing.
- Radiation therapy patients receive treatment every day, therefore, scheduling counseling sessions is easy. Patients can be seen before or after their treatment times.
- Allow 30 to 45 minutes for the initial appointment and 15 to 30 minutes for follow-ups. Follow-ups should occur every 2 to 3 weeks or weekly in high risk patients, such as those with head and neck cancer.
- Follow-up visits can be beneficial after treatment is completed, especially in the head and neck population. These patients frequently lose weight for months after completing treatment due to the long-lasting side effects of treatment (14).

Assessment Considerations with Radiation Therapy Patients

Initial consult. This should include diet history or current intake, weight history, any current nutrition-related problems and a determination of baseline nutrition status. Common side effects should be discussed and specific suggestions given even if the patient currently has no problems.

Restrictive therapeutic diets i.e. diabetic or low fat/cholesterol. These can be relaxed during radiation therapy treatment if oral intake is compromised.

Medications. These are helpful in managing the side effects of treatment. Knowledge of frequently prescribed medications and the schedule and form of these medications is important. See Appendix B for further information on common medications.

Patient education. Written material should be provided for each patient. The information should be written clearly and simply. The Oncology Nutrition Dietetic Practice Group developed and field-tested patient education materials which are available for purchase (The American Dietetic Association, 800/877-1600 ext. 5000). Breast cancer patients usually do not have problems related to radiation therapy, but may need information on low fat, high fiber, and weight maintenance.

Food preparation/availability. Encourage patients to keep easy-to-eat foods such as single portions of canned fruit, yogurt, pudding, or packaged crackers handy at all times, especially on days when they have appointments with their physicians or expect to be away from home for a prolonged period of time. If the patient lives far from the treatment facility and needs to occupy temporary housing, it can be difficult to meet nutrition needs, especially a patient staying in a hotel without cooking facilities. Making milkshakes or eating often could be difficult under these circumstances.

Supplements. Provide a variety of samples of nutrition supplements, i.e. liquids, puddings, powders, bars. A list of stores that carry these products and community resources to help patients with limited financial resources is helpful. Arnold and Richter found that nutrition supplements increase calorie and protein intake rather than displace these nutrients in usual food intake (15).

Calorie and protein requirements. These are dependent on the type of cancer, the treatment the patient is currently receiving, and nutrition status, in addition to age and gender. See Chapter 4, *Calorie, Protein, Fluid, and Micronutrient Requirements of the Oncology Patient,* for further information.

Enteral feedings. These may be needed in patients unable to consume an adequate diet. Head and neck cancer patients frequently need enteral nutrition support to maintain weight. Numerous studies demonstrate the benefit of enteral feeding initiated at the onset of treatment before significant weight loss has occurred (7,8,16,17). See chapter 11 on enteral nutrition for further information.

Total parenteral nutrition (TPN). This is rarely used in the radiation therapy area, as most patients are able to be fed orally or enterally (18). However, patients with severe radiation enteritis may require TPN. Pharmacologic and nutrition therapy are used in the acute radiation enteritis patient, whereas surgical treatment may be used in the chronic radiation enteritis patient to manage small bowel obstruction or perforation (19). See chapter 12 on parenteral nutrition for further information.

Medical Nutrition Therapy in the Radiation Therapy Patient

Nutrition care of the cancer patient should support positive nutrition status, adequate body composition, maintenance of functional status, and quality of life. During cancer treatment, patients should be provided a nutritious diet (20). Several important benefits of good nutrition include:
• Patients who maintain good nutrition status are more likely to tolerate treatment side effects (21).
• A healthy diet helps patients maintain their strength during treatment (21).
• Adequate nutrition prevents body tissues from breaking down and allows rebuilding of tissues harmed by the cancer treatment (21).
• Patients who do not consume adequate calories use stored nutrients as an energy source, which may lead to protein wasting, weight loss and an increased risk of infection (22).

Cancer treatment side effects vary from patient to patient and are affected by many factors, including nutrition status prior to treatment, part of the body being treated, length and type of treatment, and dose of treatment. Also, many patients experience a loss of appetite or nausea during treatment due to depression and anxiety about their disease and how it will impact their future. During this time, the health professional should assess the patient's nutritional status and provide recommendations for each patient, as symptoms and preferences vary.

Table 7.2 offers suggestions to help overcome the variety of symptoms that are typical for many cancer patients and that relate specifically to the radiation therapy patient. The tips are intended to reinforce information provided by other health care professionals for the patient's diet plan during the treatment. (See Appendix A for tips for managing nutrition-related problems, as well as ideas to increase calorie and protein intake.)

Table 7.2   Management of Nutrition-Related Side Effects (20–22)

Side Effect	Suggestions for the Patient
Thick saliva / dry mouth	Use salt and soda mouthwash (1 tsp.salt and 1 tsp. baking soda to 1 qt. water) before meals and snacks, and during the day.
	Eat starchy foods (rice, noodles, bread, potatoes) with gravy, sauce: soften foods by dunking in beverages (coffee, milk, soups).
	To decrease risk of dental caries, avoid candies or gum that contain sugar; try sugar free gum or candy instead.
	Try sour foods such as lemons, limes, or grapefruit to increase saliva production; however, this may cause pain if mouth or throat is sore.
	Carry water or fluids with you at all times; take sips often.
	Ask a physician if artificial saliva is appropriate.
	Use a humidifier at home, especially at night, to reduce dry-mouth symptoms.
	Avoid alcohol, tobacco, commercial mouthwashes, and liquid vitamin-mineral supplements that contain alcohol.
	Avoid smoking.

continued

Side Effect	Suggestions for the Patient
Taste changes or loss of taste	Look for foods with a stronger taste (i.e. chocolate is stronger than vanilla).
	Try unusual combinations, (eg, pickle juice milkshakes have been known to combat sweet intolerance).
	Try tart or spicy foods unless the mouth or throat is sore.
	Smell foods and try to remember how they tasted before treatment.
	Use plastic silverware to reduce a metallic taste.
	Try cold or cool-temperature foods that have less taste or aroma.
	Try nutrition supplements intended for tube feeding; these are usually unflavored and can be better tolerated if sweet tastes are a problem.
	Look at area of tongue receiving radiation. Patient may still be able to taste certain flavors if only part of tongue is receiving radiation.
Dysphagia	Keep jars of gravy or sauces at home to add to foods to increase moisture.
	Eat blended foods; warm foods before blending for best results. Commercially prepared baby foods may also help.
	Realize nutrition supplements or milkshake recipes are frequently necessary for a majority of calorie and protein intake.
	Avoid alcohol, tobacco, and spices.
Diarrhea	Avoid raw fruits and vegetables, whole grain bread and cereals, nuts, popcorn, skins, seeds, legumes, and other vegetables with hulls; avoid gas-producing foods.
	Try pectin-containing foods like potatoes, applesauce, oatmeal, bananas, cooked carrots, and rice; they act as a thickening agent for stool formation.
	Avoid large quantities of fruit juice and sweetened fruit drinks because they may increase osmotic diarrhea.
	Replace fluid losses with 1 cup of water for each episode of diarrhea.
	Consider elemental oral nutrition supplements or those containing MCT oil if fat malabsorption appears to be a problem.
	Avoid or limit caffeine daily intake to no more than 2 to 3 servings of regular coffee, tea, or cola beverages.
	Ask a physician if medications are appropriate.
Gas and bloating	Avoid gas-producing foods such as broccoli, cabbage, cauliflower, beans, lentils, onions, garlic, beer, carbonated beverages, and eggs.
	Use an enzyme product (eg, Beano®) to help digest the carbohydrate in gas-producing foods.
	Eat five to six small meals a day. Do not skip meals; do not overeat.
Nausea	Schedule a light meal before or after treatment and/or carry food with you to eat after treatment.
	Consult a social worker if symptoms occur immediately before or after treatment; these may be due to stress.
	Ask physician if medications are appropriate.
Vomiting	If vomiting occurs in conjunction with coughing (eg, patient with lung cancer), medication may be required to reduce coughing.
	If vomiting is due to gagging (eg, patient with head and neck cancer), liquid foods may be best tolerated and hot liquids can cut phlegm. Ask a physician if medication can help.

continued

Side Effect	Suggestions for the Patient
Sore mouth and throat	Try buttermilk; it can be soothing when used as a mouth rinse.
	Consider liquid or pureed foods for the majority of the treatment.
	Consider nutrition supplements and milkshake recipes for the majority of calorie and protein intake if unable to consume solid foods in adequate quantities.
	Try nectars instead of apple, grape, or acidic juices.
	Try sucking on ice or popsicles prior to eating.
	Ask physician about use of medication to numb throat and mouth.
Fat malabsorption	Ask a physician about the use of pancreatic enzymes (ie, patients with pancreatic cancer or insufficiency). Enzymes need to be taken with meals and snacks.
	Use MCT oil if necessary. The dietetics professional can supply recipes for its use.
	Try a low-fat diet while maintaining adequate calorie intake if pancreatic enzymes do not help.

Sources:
Kelly K. An overview on how to nourish the cancer patient by mouth. *Ca.* 1986; 58:1897-1901.

Darbinian JA, Coulston AM. *Impact of Radiation Therapy on the Nutrition Status of the Cancer Patient: Acute and Chronic Complications.* In Bloch AS, ed. Nutrition Management of the Cancer Patient. Rockville, Maryland: Aspen Publications; 1990: 192–197.

Eating Hints-Recipes and Tips for Better Nutrition During Cancer Treatment. Washington, DC: US Department of Health and Human Services, National Institutes of Health; 1998. NIH Publication 98-2079.

Summary

Patients may have many nutrition problems due to the side effects of radiation therapy. A dietetics professional can help maximize intake and improve quality of life by managing nutrition-related side effects of therapy. Therefore, the dietetics professional should market medical nutrition therapy services to radiation therapy programs and become a vital team member of the multidisciplinary team. Weight loss does not need to be a side effect of treatment.

Glossary of Terms Relating to Radiation Therapy

choleretic enteropathy excessive excretion of bile

dysgeusia impairment or perversion of the gustatory sense such that normal tastes are interpreted as being unpleasant or completely different

dysomia distortion of normal smell perception

dysphagia inability to swallow or difficulty in swallowing

fractionation to separate into fractions

mucositis inflammation of a mucous membrane, frequently refers to oral cavity

odynophagia pain upon swallowing

trismus contraction of the muscles of mastication

xerostomia dryness of the mouth caused by the arresting of normal salivary secretion

References

1. Washington CM, Leaver DT. Introduction to Radiation Therapy Vol. 1. St Louis, Mo: Mosby-Year Book; 1996.
2. Donaldson SS, Lenon RA. Alterations of nutritional status: impact of chemotherapy and radiation therapy. *Cancer*. 1979;43:2036-2052.
3. Donaldson SS. Nutritional consequences of radiotherapy. *Cancer Research*. 1977;37:2407-2413.
4. Polisena CG, Carr-Davis E, Edmondson M, Unpublished data, The Cleveland Clinic Foundation, 1997.
5. Lopez MJ, Robinson P, Madden T, Highbarger T. Nutritional support and prognosis in patients with head and neck cancer. *J Surg Oncology*. 1994;55:33-36.
6. Daly JM, Durbrick SJ, Copeland EM. Evaluation of nutritional indices as prognostic indicators in the cancer patient. *Cancer*. 1979;43:925-931.
7. Pezner RD, Archambeau JO, Lipsett JA, Kokal WA, Thayer W, Hill LR. Tube feeding enteral nutritional support in patients receiving radiation therapy for advanced head and neck cancer. *Int J Radiat Oncology Biol Phys*. 1987;13:935-939.
8. Daly JM, Hearne B, Dunaj F, LePorte B, Vikram B, Strong E, Green M, Muggio F, Groshen S, DeCosse JJ. Nutritional rehabilitation in patients with advanced head and neck cancer receiving radiation therapy. *Am J Surg*. 1984;148:514-520.
9. Polisena CG. Outcome of radiation therapy patients' perception of benefit of medical nutrition therapy received during treatment. *J Am Diet Assoc*. 1997;97(suppl):A-26. Abstract.
10. Blackburn GL, Bistrian BR, Maine BS, Schlamm HT, Smith MF. Nutritional and metabolic assessment of the hospitalized patient. *JPEN*. 1977;1:11-22.
11. Chencharick JD, Mossman KL. Nutritional consequences of the radiotherapy of head and neck cancer. *Cancer*. 1983;51:811-815.
12. Johnston CA, Keane TJ, Prudo SM. Weight loss in patients receiving radical radiation therapy for head and neck cancer: a prospective study. *JPEN*. 1982;6:399-402.
13. Brown JK. Gender, age, usual weight, and tobacco use as predictors of weight loss in patients with lung cancer. *Oncol Nurs Forum*. 1993;20:466-472.
14. Backstrom I, Funegard U, Andersson I, Franzen L, Johansson I. Dietary intake in head and neck irradiated patients with permanent dry mouth symptoms. *Oral Oncol, Eur J Cancer*. 1995;31:253-257.
15. Arnold C, Richter MP. The effect of oral nutritional supplements on head and neck cancer. *Int J Radiat Oncology Biol Phys*. 1989;16:1595-1599.
16. Tyldesley S, Sheehan F, Munk P, Tsang V, Skargard D, Bowman CA, Hobenshield SE. The use of radiologically placed gastrostomy tubes in head and neck cancer patients receiving radiotherapy. *Int J Radiat Oncology Biol Phys*. 1996;36:1205-1209.
17. Hearne BE, Dunaj JM, Daly JM, Strong EW, Vikram B, LePorte BJ, DeCosse JJ. Enteral nutrition support in head and neck cancer: tube vs. oral feeding during radiation therapy. *J Am Dietet Assoc*. 1985;85:669-667.
18. Hill ADK, Daly JM. Current indications for intravenous nutritional support in oncology patients. *Surg Oncol Clin N Am*. 1995;4:549-563.
19. Meek AG. The clinical syndrome of radiation enteritis. RD. 1996; 16 (spring): 1-4,15.
20. Shils, ME. Nutrition and diet in cancer management. In: Shils M, Olson, Shike, eds. *Modern Nutrition in Health and Disease*. Philadelphia, Pa: Lippincott;1994:1317-1347.
21. PDQ: the National Cancer Institute's computerized database. Bethesda, MD: National Cancer Institute; date unknown; cited 1998 Feb 9. Available from: http://cancernet.nci.nih.gov/clindq/supportive/Nutrition_Physician.html.
22. Ottery FD. Definition of standardized nutritional assessment and interventional pathways in oncology. *Nutrition*. 1996;12(suppl):15S-19S.

Additional Reading

Gastorf, L, Vanderzyl, J. Nutritional support during radiotherapy. *Dimensions Oncol Nurs.* 1991; 5:17-20.

Hunter AMB. Clinical observation. Nutrition management of patients with neoplastic disease of the head and neck treated with radiation therapy. *Nutr Clin Practice.* 1996; 11: 157-169.

Klien, S, Koretz, RL. Nutrition support in patients with cancer; what do the data really show? *Nutr Clin Practice* 1994; 9:91-100.

Weihofen, D. *The Cancer Survival Cookbook.* Minneapolis, MN: Chronimed Publishing; 1998.

8

Nutrition Implications of Surgical Oncology

Ginny Allison MS, RD, CNSD

Barbara Eldridge, RD

Christine Polisena MS, MBA, RD

Teresa Dixon RD, CNSD

Rashida Jinnah MS, RD, CNSD

Surgery, the primary treatment modality for many cancers, can affect the body by mechanical and physiological alteration. The immediate metabolic response to surgery in cancer patients is similar to those who have surgery for benign disease. Commonly experienced side effects include fatigue, increased calorie and protein needs for wound healing, and temporary alterations in appetite and bowel function secondary to anesthesia and analgesia.

Cancer patients often have significant weight loss prior to surgery, due to disease and/or other treatment. Consequently there is greater incidence of postoperative morbidity and mortality. It is often necessary to provide enteral or parenteral nutrition support perioperatively. Surgeries of the alimentary tract have specific nutritional sequel depending on the site.

Head and Neck Cancer

Common alterations in head and neck cancer, secondary to the tumor and/or surgical intervention(s), may alter the ability to speak, chew, swallow, smell, taste, and/or see. These alterations create unique needs and should be managed with a multidisciplinary team approach. The most common types of carcinomas arising in the areodigestive tract are of squamous cell origin. Table 8.1 lists the common postsurgical complications in this population (1,2). Table 8.2 offers solutions to the postsurgical complications of head and neck surgery (1,2). The use of postoperative enteral feedings is common.

Patients should be screened upon initial assessment for possible coexisting complications such as alcoholism. Appropriate medical nutrition therapy should follow (see Chapter 2, *Patient-Generated Subjective Global Assessment;* Appendix A, *Management of Nutrition-Related Symptoms;* Chapter 13, *Pharmacological Management of Anorexia and Cachexia;* and Appendix B, *Common Supportive Drug Therapies Used in Oncology*). Management of coexisting complications of the head and neck cancer patient are outlined in Table 8.3 (1,2). Head and neck cancer treatment may entail surgery, radiation, chemotherapy, or combinations thereof (see Chapter 6, *Chemotherapy and Nutrition Implications,* and Chapter 7, *Nutrition Concerns with the Radiation Therapy Patient*).

Table 8.1   Common Postsurgical Complications: Head and Neck Cancer Surgeries

Surgery	Compromised Swallowing and Aspiration Potential	Delayed Swallowing (more than 10 seconds)	Dysphagia, Odynophagia, Postoperative Swelling	Dental Extraction/ Altered Dentition	Dry Mouth, Altered Taste	Inability to Meet Calorie Needs
Base of tongue Resection	X		X			X
Total glossectomy		X	X			X
Partial glossectomy	X		X			
Floor of mouth resection		X	X	X		X
Hypopharyngeal resection	X	X	X			X
Total laryngectomy		X	X			X
Partial laryngectomy	X		X			X
Total maxillectomy	X		X			X
Pharyngo-laryngectomy		X	X			X
CRP resection			X	X		X
Oropharyngeal resection	X	X	X	X		X
Nasopharyngeal resection		X	X	X		X
Mandibulectomy			X	X	X	X
Buccal/Mucosal resection			X	X	X	
Any procedure involving loss of 7th cranial nerve	X	X				X
Neck dissection						
Auricular resection						
Orbital resection Parotidectomy					X	
Rhinectomy						
Thyroidectomy			X		X	

Table 8.2   Postsurgical Complications due to Functional Alterations After Head and Neck Surgery: Solutions

Postsurgical Complication	Solutions
Compromised swallowing and aspiration potential	Avoid sticky, bulky, thin foods and foods that crumble. Use thickening agent. Adhere to pureed thick liquid diet. Use supplemental tube feeding if unable to consume > 60% of daily needs.
Delayed swallowing—more than 10 seconds	Mandatory nasogastric tube feeding first 10 to 21 days; can usually begin oral diet at 10 days if palatal drop[1] present
Placement of obturator[2] or palatal drop prosthesis[1]	Full liquid and pureed foods allowed after packing is removed 2 to 3 days after surgery
Dental extractions	Food texture modification Assessment of long-term dental prognosis with appropriate instruction for texture alteration; recipes for home, mouth and dental care management Feedback to and from dental team regarding dentures
Dysphagia, odynophagia, postoperative swelling	Foods—moist to pureed, depending upon pain/ swelling Avoid highly spiced, acidic, and abrasive foods Use liquid supplement shakes
Dry mouth/altered taste	Frequent liquids—emphasis on calorie/protein content Soft/moist meals Avoid dry foods. Zinc sulfate lozenges for altered taste; recommended dosage: 45 mg zinc sulfate TID (3) Dental and mouth care management
Inability to meet calorie needs and/or malnourished prior to surgery	Perioperative enteral feedings (see Chapter 11) Parenteral nutrition if gut nonfunctioning (see Chapter 12)

[1]A removable bridge that fits contour of palate; reduces palatal height to enable food mastication and speech in patients with speech and dental impairment.
[2]Synthetic customized removable device of varying form and function. In the head and neck cancer patient, used to aid speech and swallowing.

Table 8.3   Common Coexisting Complications in the Head and Neck Surgical Patient: Interventions

Complication	Nutrition Implication	Intervention
I. Alcoholism	1. Malnutrition due to disproportionate alcohol/nutrient intake 2. Nutrient malabsorption of B_{12}, folic acid, ascorbic acid, thiamin, Mg, zinc 3. Glucose intolerance due to pancreatic inflammation	1. Assess feasibility of feeding tube placement with weight <80% IBW or <90% UBW 2. Supplementation daily (See Chapter 4 for replacement guidelines) 3. NPO/TPN if acute pancreatitis (see Chapter 12 for TPN guidelines in pancreatitis), Insulin as needed
II. Cirrhosis of the liver	1. Altered utilization of macronutrients 2. Steatorrhea	1. Nonencephalopathic: Increased calorie (1.5–1.75 × BEE) Increased protein (1.5/kg dry wt) Encephalopathic: Protein restrict to 0.5 g/kg dry wt High biological value/branched Chain amino acid protein source Calories (1.2–1.5 × BEE) (4,5) 2. IV or IM, vitamin supplementation of B vitamins, thiamine and fat-soluble (See Chapter 4 for guidelines)
III. Chyle fistula	Nutrient needs up to 3 x BEE	1. Low-fat diet or formula <10 g/fat per day 2. Medium chain triglyceride oil formula or supplementation 3. If drainage not controlled with above restriction: NPO/TPN (see Chapter 12 for TPN guidelines)
IV. Chemotherapy or Radiation therapy	1. Cachexia, anorexia, mucositis, enteritis, nausea, vomiting, bowel alterations 2. Delayed wound healing	1. See Chapters 6, 7, and 13 for guidelines 2. If chemo/XRT to be repeated every 3 to 4 weeks enteral or parenteral nutrition indicated
V. Specific food group avoidance: distaste for meats; lactose intolerance; omission of vegetables, grains; fiber intolerance	1. Inadequate protein, calorie intake 2. Vitamin/mineral deficiencies 3. Constipation 4. Diarrhea	1. Protein alternatives/powders 2. Lactose free milk, milk alternatives, lactaid pills, liquid supplements 3. Vitamin supplementation (see Chapter 4) 4. Zinc sulfate tablets 45 mg TID (3) 5. Education: cooking, recipes, texture alteration 6. Fiber supplement, bowel regimen

Gastrointestinal Cancers

Esophageal Cancer

Surgical intervention has reduced mortality and morbidity rates for esophageal cancer. Aggressive surgery has also provided palliation of dysphagia and increased longevity compared to other therapy. Surgical treatment consists of removing the diseased portion of esophagus. Figures 8.1a, 8.1b, and 8.1c depict standard procedures for esophagogastrectomy, based on location of the tumor. Use of jejunostomy tube feedings for 10 to 14 days postoperative is common in this population. Gastrostomies may not be indicated in this patient population if the esophageal surgery involves the distal esophagus and the gastro-esophageal junction (lower esophageal sphincter) is altered or surgically removed. Refer to Tables 8.4 and 8.5 for the common postsurgical complications and nutrition interventions (6).

Figure 8.1a   Transhiatal approach (esophagectomy without thoracotomy). **A,** upper midline and left cervical incision; **B,** extent of resection (shaded area); **C,** completed anastomosis.

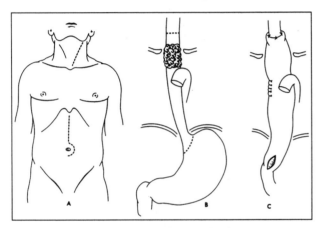

Reprinted with permission from Ellis FH Jr. Esophagogastrectomy for carcinoma: technical considerations based on anatomic location of lesion. *Surg Clin North Am.* 1980;60:273.

Figure 8.1b   Esophagogastrectomy with thoracoabdominal approach. **A,** combined abdominal incision and right thoracotomy for lesions of the upper thoracic esophagus; **B,** extent of resection (shaded area); **C1,** esophagogastrostomy in the chest; **C2,** if submucosal spread is great, cervical anastomosis can be performed through a third incision.

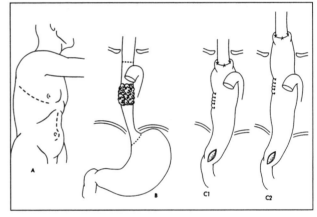

Reprinted with permission from Ellis FH Jr. Esophagogastrectomy for carcinoma: technical considerations based on anatomic location of lesion. *Surg Clin North Am.* 1980;60:273.

Figure 8.1c   Technique of esophagogastrectomy and esophagogastrostomy for carcinoma of the cardia. **A,** site of incision; **B,** extent of resection (shaded area); **C,** completed esophagogastrostomy.

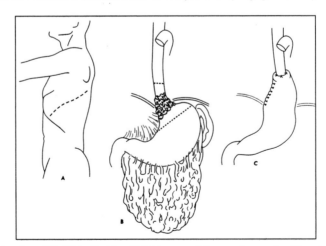

Reprinted with permission from Ellis HF Jr, Shahlan DM. Tumors of the esophagus. In: Glenn WWL, Baue AE, Geha AS, Hammon GL, Laks H (ed.). *Thoracic and Cardiovascular Surgery,* 4th ed. Norwalk: Conn: Appleton & Lange, 1983.

Gastric Cancer

Surgical intervention is the only effective curative therapy in the primary treatment of gastric cancer. It is a common approach for palliation as well. Surgical options include distal subtotal gastrectomy, proximal subtotal gastrectomy, or total gastrectomy. The gastrointestinal tract is maintained by anastamosis of
- the small intestine to the gastric remnant
- distal stomach to the esophagus
- small intestine to esophagus (with or without jejunal reservoirs) (Figure 8.2).

Refer to Tables 8.4 and 8.5 for surgical complications and nutrition interventions (6).

Figure 8.2   Surgical Resections and Reconstruction for the Three Locations of Gastric Cancer. Left to right: Distal Gastrectomy, Proximal Gastrectomy, Total Gastrectomy (method of reconstruction shown below each procedure).

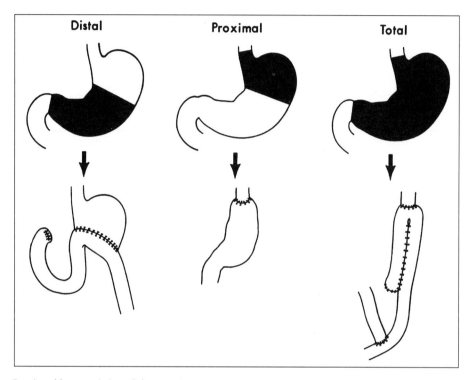

Reprinted by permission of the American Cancer Society, Inc.

Table 8.4   Common Postsurgical Complications: Gastrointestinal Surgeries

Surgery	Gastro-paresis	Fat malab-sorption	Hyper-glycemia	Hypertri-glyceri-demia	Encepha-lopathy	Fluid/Electrolyte imbalance	Anasto-motic level	Chyle leak	Dumping syndrome	Vitamin malab-sorption	Mineral malab-sorption
Esopha-gogastric	X					X	X	X	X		
Gastric	X	X	X						X	B_{12},D	Fe,Ca
Pancreas	X	X	X			X		X		A,D,E,K,B_{12}	Ca,Fe,Zn
Hepato-cellular			X	X	X	X		X		A,D,E,K,B_1, Folic acid	Mg,Zn, Restrict Cu,Mn
Gallbladder	X	X	X			X		X		B_{12},A,D,E,K	Ca,Fe,Zn
Bile duct	X	X	X			X		X		B_{12},A,D,E,K	Ca,Fe,Zn
Small bowel	X	X	X			X		X		B_{12},A,D,E,K	Ca,Fe,Zn
Colorectal						X				B_{12}	Na,K, Mg,Ca

Table 8.5   Postsurgical Complications due to Functional and Absorptive Alterations after GI Surgery: Interventions

Postsurgical Complications	Interventions
Gastroparesis Gastric stasis Gastric reflux	A gastrostomy tube (GT) is placed for drainage of stomach contents. With improvement in gastric motility, the patient tolerates the tube being clamped. The diet is advanced from clear liquids to six regular small feedings. The patient is discharged on a regular diet, six small meals and maybe a tube feeding at night. Tube feeding is continued until a patient is able to meet 70%–75% of assessed nutrition requirements by PO intake alone. Feeding jejunostomy tube (JT) is placed during surgery. Tube feeding is started post-op and advanced per tolerance of the patient. Formula selection is dependent on type of surgery. For esophageal and gastric cancer, a polymeric high protein formula is used. For pancreas, duodenal, bile duct and gall bladder surgeries, a low-fat, glutamine-containing formula is used secondary to anticipation of fat malabsorption and maintenance of GI tract, ie, decreasing mucosal injury post a lengthy operative procedure which is most often proceeded by chemotherapy and radiation. Tube feeding is changed to an isotonic low long chain triglyceride (high medium chain triglycerides) formula prior to discharge. (5,10,14) Oral intake guidelines: • Small frequent meals • Foods with high caloric density • Keep head and shoulders elevated above stomach after eating • Avoid tight clothing around the waist
Fat malabsorption	Pancreatic lipase is needed for the hydrolysis of most dietary fat. Ninety percent of pancreatic function can be lost without interfering with fat breakdown and subsequent malabsorption. Oral pancreatic enzyme replacement can partially correct pancreatic insufficiency, so dietary restriction of fat may not be necessary. MCT absorption occurs without hydrolysis with pancreatic lipase and hence the choice of tube feeding formula. Fat malabsorption due to decreased secretion of bile salts is treated with a low fat diet and use of MCT oil (5).
Hyperglycemia	Conventional dietary restrictions may need to be liberalized to achieve adequate caloric intake. Hyperglycemia should be controlled by an oral hypoglycemic agent and/or insulin.
Hypertriglyceridemia	Avoid overfeeding, recommend 25–35 kcals/kg body weight. Limit IV lipids (14).
Hepatic encephalopathy	Provide adequate protein to facilitate hepatic cell nutrition without excess production of ammonia from endogenous and exogenous protein catabolism, 1–1.2 grams/kg dry weight. In the presence of encephalopathy, 0.5 g/kg dry weight. Up to 1.5 g/kg dry weight if using branched chain amino acids (4,5).

Fluid and electrolyte balance	• Increased fluid needs secondary to: nasogastric/gastrostomy losses; diarrhea
	• Decreased fluid needs secondary to ascites.
	• Increased electrolyte needs: sodium, potassium, magnesium, and zinc secondary to: duodenal resection; diarrhea
	• Decreased electrolyte needs:
	  Sodium if ascites is present.
	  Decrease needs for copper and manganese in hepatic failure.

Anastomic leak/breakdown	Will require full nutrition support via jejunostomy tube or TPN (if no enteral access available)
Chyle leak (if thoracic duct or lymph accidentally nicked during surgery)	• Minimal to no fat by mouth/enterally • Enteral feedings with minimal fat • Consider MCT supplementation - absorbable form of fat (bypass lymphatic absorption) • May require TPN
Dumping syndrome (Although variable, seen in either subtotal or more commonly total gastrectomy)	Antidumping Diet: • Avoid hyperosmolar feedings (low simple carbohydrates) • High protein, high complex carbohydrates • Small frequent meals • Liquids between solid meals • Foods high in pectin may be helpful (apples, bananas, oatmeal, rice potatoes) in reducing transit time • Encourage patient to eat slowly in a relaxed atmosphere • Use of long analog of somatostatin
Vitamins	• Fat soluble vitamin supplements to compensate for malabsorption from steatorrhea • Monitor for B12 deficiency if ileal absorption is in question • Intramuscular B12 every month required for patient after gastrectomies and pancreaticoduodenectomies • Thiamin and folic acid replacement for patients with hepatocellular cancer • Vitamin D supplementation postgastrectomy
Minerals	• Calcium: decreased calcium absorption secondary to duodenum bypass may need calcium supplementation especially in postmenopausal women. • Calcium oxalate stones can develop after surgery for colorectal cancer. Encourage increased fluid intake. Restrict high-oxalate foods if needed. • Monitor for metabolic bone disease, postgastrectomy can be treated with vitamin D and calcium. • Increase needs of magnesium and zinc with the use of diuretics, ie, Furosemide

Pancreatic Cancer

Pancreatic cancer is the second most common visceral malignancy and fifth leading cause of cancer mortality in the United States (10). Cigarette smoking, high-fat diets, ingestion of meat, and total calorie intake, especially when derived from carbohydrates, dairy products, and seafood have been associated with the development of pancreatic cancer (8,9,10). Surgery offers the best chance of a "cure" in pancreatic malignancy. The Whipple procedure or a pancreaticoduodenectomy is performed (Figure 8.3) (7,8,9). The use of a jejumostomy tube feeding for 4 to 6 weeks postoperatively is common (10). Refer to Tables 8.4 and 8.5 for common postsurgical complications and nutrition interventions.

Figure 8.3   Pancreaticoduodenectomy.

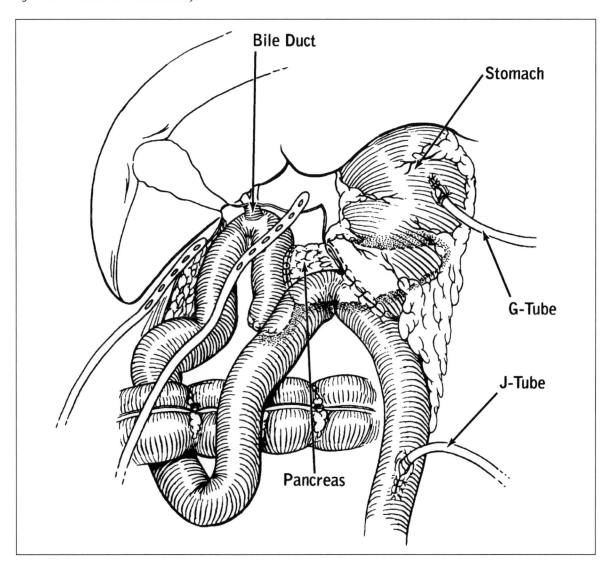

Source: Pancreatic Tumor Study Group, M. D. Anderson Cancer Center, University of Texas. Reprinted with permission.

Liver Cancer

Hepatocellular carcinoma is the most common type of primary liver cancer (11). Other types of "malignant" liver tumors include angiosarcomas, cholangiocarcinomas, and hepatoblasotmas in children. Risk factors include hepatitis B infection, alcohol-induced cirrhosis, aflatoxin contaminated food and certain drugs. The liver is also the most common site of metastasis. Surgical resection of liver cancer often requires removal of significant liver tissue. Surgical resection of metastatic lesions is beneficial in patients with colorectal cancer and Wilm's tumor when there are ≤4 metastatic tumors present. Refer to Tables 8.4 and 8.5 for common postsurgical complications and nutrition interventions (7,9,12).

Carcinoma of the Gall Bladder

Gallbladder cancer incidence is the seventh most common type of GI cancer in the United States and is treated surgically by cholecystectomy, liver resection, lymphadenectomy, and/or hepatojejunostomy (11). Surgical implications and nutrition interventions are similar to pancreas and hepatocellular cancer. Refer to Tables 8.4 and 8.5 for the common postsurgical complications and nutrition interventions used (7,9,12).

Carcinoma of the Bile Duct (Cholangiocarcinoma)

Cancer of the bile duct or cholangiocarcinoma is relatively uncommon in the United States (11). It is surgically treated with a pancreaticoduodenectomy. Surgical implication and nutrition interventions are similar to patients with pancreatic cancer. Refer to Tables 8.4 and 8.5 for common postsurgical complications and nutrition interventions (7,9, 12).

Cancer of the Small Bowel

Cancers of the small bowel are uncommon. The primary cancers of the small bowel are duodenal, leiomyoma, and leiomyosarcoma. The small bowel is not susceptible to carcinogens, but metastatic disease originating from melanoma, lymph, breast, cervix, and kidney can occur (7,9,12).

Cancer of the jejuneum and ileum are usually treated by resection. Side effects depend on length of resection and ability of the small bowel to adapt. Degree of malabsorption increases with the length of resection. Jejunal resections result in hyperplasia of the ileum and assumption of proximate absorptive functions except jejunal enterohormone secretions. Ileal resection greater than 100 cm and/or loss of ileocecal valve results in steatorrhea and impaired vitamin B_{12} absorption (5). Patients must follow a diet for 6 to 8 weeks after surgery that avoids food such as nuts, seeds, skins, popcorn, raw fruits, raw vegetables, dried fruits, and other foods that increase risk for obstruction. Surgical implications and nutrition interventions are similar to pancreaticoduodenectomy. Refer to Tables 8.4 and 8.5 for common postsurgical complications and nutrition interventions used.

Colorectal Cancer

The primary therapy for colon and rectal cancer is surgery. Conventional surgical procedures for colorectal cancer are noted in Figure 8.4. Colostomies are created following procedures where a portion of the colon is removed, and a remnant of the colon is brought through the abdominal wall. Ileostomies are created when there is surgical removal of the terminal ileum, ileal-cecal juncture, colon, and anus. A remnant of the ileum is brought through the abdominal wall to create the ileostomy. An alternative procedure is ileal reservoir after proctocolectomy which allows for daily normal resumption of colonic functions. Both colostomies and ileostomies can be temporary or permanent.

Ostomies can promote high losses of fluid and electrolytes, which is usually related to location of the ostomy and functional ability of the remaining GI tract. Ileostomies cause greater losses of fluid because the colon is bypassed (major site of fluid absorption). Output may also be excessive with macronutrient malabsorption. Colostomies may have little effect on stool output if much of the colon is still functional; ileostomies, on the other hand, can be expected to produce more liquid consistency stool. A diet eliminating food such as nuts, skins, seeds, popcorn, raw fruits, raw vegetables, dried fruits, and other foods that increase risk for obstruction is used postoperatively for 6 to 8 weeks. Refer to Tables 8.4 and 8.5 for common postoperative complications and nutrition interventions (13).

Figure 8.4   Surgical Resections of the Colon and Rectum. **A,** right hemicolectomy; **B,** extended right hemicolectomy; **C,** transverse colectomy; **D,** left hemicolectomy; **E,** sigmoid resection; **F,** rectosigmoid resection

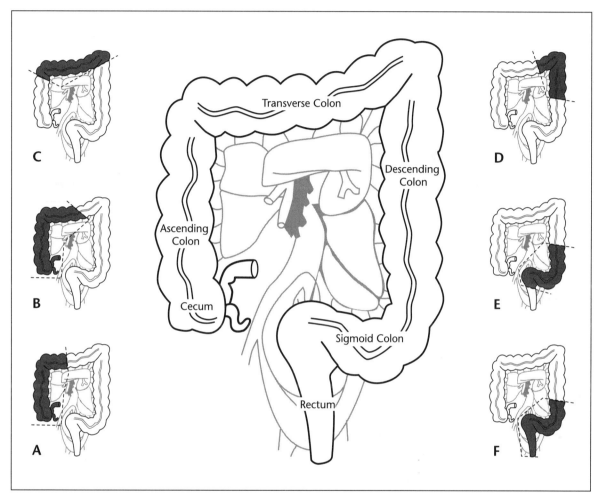

Adapted with permission from Ellis FH Jr. Esophagogastrectomy for carcinoma: technical considerations based on anatomic location of lesion. *Surg Clin North Am.* 1980;60:273.

Alteration of Nutrient Absorption Secondary to Surgical Resection

In addition to functional alterations secondary to resection of the GI tract, nutrient absorption is also compromised. Tables 8.4 and 8.5 provide details regarding specific nutrients that are problematic and nutrition interventions. Table 8.6 demonstrates nutrient absorption sites in the gastrointestinal tract (15).

Table 8.6   Nutrient Absorption in the Gastrointestinal Tract (15)

Nutrient	Stomach	Duodenum	Jejunum	Ileum	Colon
Water	X				X
Ethyl alcohol	X				
Calcium/Magnesium/Iron		X			
Actively absorbed monosaccharides, glucose, galactose		X	X		
Fat		X	X		
Fat soluble vitamin A and D		X	X		
Disaccharides sucorose, maltose, lactose			X		
Protein and amino acids			X	X	
Water soluble vitamins (thiamin, riboflavin, folic acid, ascorbic acid, pyridoxine)			X	X	
Vitamin B_{12}				X	
Bile salts				X	
Potassium					X
Sodium chloride					X
Short chain fatty acids and volatile fatty acids from fiber degradation					X

Additional Primary Sites/Surgeries

The surgical treatment of the following cancers does not affect the alimentary tract but patients will still have complications that will require nutrition management. Refer to Table 8.7 for a list of the types of cancers, the surgical implications, and the nutrition interventions used.

Table 8.7   Surgical Complications and Nutrition Interventions Based on Site of Cancer/Surgery

Site of Cancer/Surgery	Surgical Complications	Nutrition Interventions
Ovarian: Abdominal surgery TAH/BSO	Bloating, cramps, increase in gas Inability to meet calorie/protein needs Bowel alterations Wound healing Fatigue	Avoid gassy foods/beverages Eat nutrient dense foods that are easy to prepare Alter fiber intake to reduce gas and promote normal bowel function Assure adequate micronutrient consumption, especially vitamin C and zinc
Prostate :Prostatectomy	Incontinence Fatigue Wound healing	Adequate hydration Eat nutrient dense foods that are easily prepared Assure adequate micronutrient consumption, especially vitamin C and zinc
Breast: Mastectomy/ lumpectomy Spleen: Spleenectomy Lymph Node Dissection	Fatigue Wound healing	Eat nutrient-dense foods that are easily prepared Assure adequate micronutrient consumption, especially vitamin C and zinc
Brain: Brain surgery	Steroid-induced hyperglycemia Nausea/vomiting Decreased appetite Fatigue	Monitor blood sugar levels and avoid simple carbohydrates as necessary See Appendix A for symptom management suggestions Eat nutrient dense foods that are easily prepared Assure adequate micronutrient consumption, especially vitamin C and zinc

Summary

Surgical treatment can place oncology patients at nutrition risk due to the postsurgical complications. Knowledge of potential problems and solutions by dietetic professionals allows for proactive nutrition therapy.

References

1. McClure S. *Nutritional Management of the Head and Neck Cancer Patient*. Houston, Tx: The University of Texas M. D. Anderson Cancer Center, Department of Clinical Nutrition; 1997.

2. Kyle U. The patient with head and neck cancer. In: Block A, ed. *Nutrition Management of the Cancer Patient*. Rockville, Md: Aspen Publishers; 1990:53-64.

3. Ripamonti C, Zecca E, Brunneli C, Fulfaro F, Villa S, Balzarini A, et al: A randomized, controlled clinical trial to evaluate the effects of zinc sulfate on cancer patients with taste alterations caused by head and neck irradiation. *Cancer*. 1998;82:1938-1945.

4. Chicago Dietetic Association and South Suburban Dietetic Association. *Manual of Clinical Dietetics*. 5th ed. Chicago, Ill: American Dietetic Association; 1996:459-464.

5. Nelson JK, Moxness KE, Jensen MD, Gastineau CF. *Mayo Clinic Diet Manual: A Handbook of Nutrition Practice*. 7th ed. St Louis, Mo: Mosby-Yearbook, Inc; 1994:227, 201.

6. Block A. Nutrition Implications in Esophageal and Gastric Cancer. In: Block A, ed. *Nutrition Management of the Cancer Patient*. Rockville, MD: Aspen Publishers; 1990:73-83.

7. Berger DH, Feig BW, Furhmann GM. *The MD Anderson Surgical Oncology Handbook*. 1st ed. New York, NY: Little Brown and Company; 1995:194-224.

8. Devita V, Helman S, Rosenberg SA. *Cancer Principles and Practice Oncology*. 5th ed., Vol. 5. New York, NY: Lippincot-Raven; 1997:1128-1148.

9. Murphy GP, Lawrence W, Lenhard RE, eds. *American Cancer Society Textbooks of Clinical Oncology*. Atlanta, Ga: The American Cancer Society, Inc; 1995:251-273.

10. Jinnah R, Zook K, Fenoglio C, Lee J, Evans D. *Early Post-op Enteral Feeding after Pancreaticoduodenectomy*. Poster Presentation Nineteenth Clinical Congress ASPEN; 1995:592.

11. American Cancer Society, 1999 statistics, www.cancer.org., April 27, 1999.

12. Grant JP, Chapman G, Russell MK. Malabsorption associated with surgical procedures and its treatment. *Nutr Clin Pract*. 1996;11:43-52.

13. Hermann M. The gastrointestinal tract: small bowel and colon. In: Block, A, ed. *Nutrition Management of the Cancer Patient*. Rockville, Md: Aspen Publishers; 1990:111-124.

14. Gottschlich M, Matarese L, Shronts E. *Nutrition Support Dietetics Core Curriculum* 2nd ed. Silver Spring, Md: Aspen Publications; 1993.

15. Enloe C. The pancreas. *Nutr Today*. 1984;March/April:23.

9

Medical Nutrition Therapy in Bone Marrow Transplantation

Paula M. Charuhas, MS, RD, FADA, CNSD

The objectives of marrow transplantation are to replace the malignant or defective hematopoietic system (the production and development of blood cells) and to restore normal hematopoiesis and immunologic function (1). Treatment consists of a preparative regimen that includes cytotoxic chemotherapy to eradicate the malignant cells and may also include total body irradiation. An infusion of autologous (patient's own) or allogeneic (from a histocompatible related or unrelated donor) marrow follows. Currently, peripheral blood stem cell transplants are being used with increased frequency and umbilical cord blood transplants are being explored as alternatives to marrow transplants (2,3).

Nutrition Assessment (4,5)

The nutrition assessment should begin pre-transplant and continue throughout the transplant course. It includes a comprehensive evaluation of nutrition history, anthropometric biochemical indices, and other factors.

Nutrition History

Assess:
- Current oral and gastrointestinal symptoms including chewing and swallowing ability, mucositis and esophagitis, taste alterations, xerostomia, heartburn, nausea, vomiting, early satiety, anorexia, and changes in bowel habits
- Current dietary modifications and special diets
- Current/past use of nutritional supplements; current use and dosage of vitamin and mineral supplements, herbal preparations, and/or other alternative medicine therapies
- Food allergies or intolerances
- Prior need for tube feeding or parenteral nutrition (PN) support
- Stage of eating development and use of infant formulas in pediatric patients

Anthropometry

- Obtain measured height (length in children < 2 years of age); assess growth history in children
- Assess weight changes from pre-illness weight; determine percent of usual weight
- Calculate ideal body weight (IBW) and percent of IBW
- Determine adjusted IBW in obese patients (6): Adjusted IBW = (Actual weight – IBW) (0.25) + IBW
- Obtain arm anthropometry to evaluate somatic muscle protein and adipose reserves; skinfold measurements obtained pre-transplant provide baseline data for serial measurements
- Determine body surface area which is often used in calculating medication dosages

$$\text{Body surface area (m}^2) = \sqrt{\frac{\text{Actual weight (kg)} \times \text{height (cm)}}{60}}$$

Biochemical Indices

Obtain baseline:
- Renal parameters (creatinine, blood urea nitrogen (BUN))
- Electrolytes (sodium, potassium, magnesium, calcium, phosphorus)
- Liver enzyme profile (bilirubin, serum glutamic-oxaloacetic transaminase (SGOT), alkaline phosphatase)
- Visceral protein parameters (albumin and/or prealbumin)
- Blood lipids (cholesterol, triglyceride)

Other

- Review medical history (ie, diabetes mellitus, hyperlipidemia) and prior therapy
- Review current medications for drug-nutrient interactions
- Assess physical strength and activity level
- Assess level of pain and pain control that may interfere with oral intake

Nutrient Requirements

Energy

Energy requirements are increased early post-transplant to account for the metabolic stress induced by the preparative regimen, fever, infections, and other metabolic complications. Suggested guidelines (4, 7):

Adult:	Baseline needs	BEE × 1.3
Adult:	Stress needs	BEE* × 1.5–1.7, or 30–35 kcal/kg
Pediatric:	Baseline needs	BMR × 1.4
	(> 45 kg)	BEE × 1.4
Pediatric:	Stress needs	BMR* *× 1.6–1.8

*BEE: Harris-Benedict equation for basal energy expenditure (8)
**BMR: basal metabolic rate (9)

Protein (4)

Protein requirements are estimated to be twice the normal recommended dietary allowance (ie, 1.5 g/kg IBW for adults) to promote tissue repair after cytoreduction and to spare breakdown of lean body mass. Protein needs may be further increased with catabolic corticosteroid therapy; needs may decrease with renal or hepatic dysfunction.

Fluids

Calculations for maintenance fluid needs are as follows (10):
- < 10 kg: 100 mL/kg/ per 24 hr
- 11–20 kg: 1000 mL plus 50 mL/kg for each kg > 10 kg per 24 hr
- 21–40 kg: 1500 mL plus 20 mL for each kg > 20 kg per 24 hr
- > 40 kg: 1500 mL/m^2/24 hr

Vitamins

Intravenous vitamin recommendations, based on guidelines provided by the Nutrition Advisory Group, American Medical Association (11), include
- Provide additional vitamin C (500 mg/day ≥ 31 kg; 250 mg/day <31 kg) to promote tissue recovery via collagen biosynthesis following cytoreductive therapy (4)
- Provide vitamin K at weekly doses of 5 mg (<11 kg) to 10 mg (≥11 kg), in PN, separate from infusion of other intravenous vitamins (4)
- Recommend oral multivitamin-mineral supplement at 100% dietary reference intake (DRI), when available, and 100% recommended dietary allowance, for nutrients where a DRI is not yet available, (without iron to prevent iron overload) following discontinuation of PN, for one year post-transplant (1)

Trace Minerals

- Suggested initial PN trace mineral additives are shown in Table 9.1 (12)
- Provide additional zinc at a suggested dose of 17 mg/liter stool output during episodes of prolonged diarrhea (13)
- Remove copper and manganese from PN with persistent hyperbilirubinemia (bilirubin > 15 mg/dL) (4)

Table 9.1   Parenteral Trace Mineral Recommendations

Mineral	Adult Dose	Pediatric Dose
Zinc	2.5-4.0 mg/day	100 mcg/kg
Copper	0.5-1.5 mg/day	15-20 mcg/kg
Chromium	10-20 mcg/day	0.14-0.5 mcg/kg
Manganese	0.1-1.0 mg/day	2-10 mcg/kg

Adapted with permission from Cunningham (12).

Electrolytes

Table 9.2 outlines suggested initial PN electrolyte recommendations (12).

Table 9.2   Suggested Initial Parenteral Nutrition Electrolyte Recommendations*

Calcium gluconate	8 mEq
Magnesium sulfate	16 mEq
Potassium chloride	25 mEq
Potassium phosphate	15 mEq
Sodium chloride	30 mEq

*Standard electrolyte additives per liter of PN solution
Adapted with permission from Cunningham (12).

Nutrition Support

Oral Feedings

Most transplant centers restrict foods high in bacterial content to decrease the risk of food-related infections. The degree of modification, however, varies. An example of a diet for immunosuppressed marrow transplant patients is presented in Box 9.1.

Enteral Feedings

Enteral feedings have been used with limited success early post-transplant due to gastrointestinal dysfunction associated with regimen-related toxicities, thrombocytopenia, and neutropenia. Issues surrounding optimum time for initiation of feedings, enteral access routes, administration methods, and appropriate formulas need to be further explored.

Parenteral Nutrition

Parenteral nutrition is generally included as standard supportive care because of the adverse oral and gastrointestinal manifestations associated with intense cytoreductive therapy. Carbohydrate, in the form of dextrose, typically comprises 50% to 60% of total calories, however, administration must be individualized (1). A lower dextrose PN concentration, coupled with intravenous lipid infusions to balance substrates, is indicated for glucose intolerance. Protein, in the form of crystalline amino acids, usually comprises 15% to 20% of total calories. Specialized pediatric amino acid formulas may be used for very young transplant patients. Lipids typically comprise 10% to 30% of total calories. For pediatric patients, the maximum lipid dosage is 4 g/kg/day (14).

Box 9.1   Diet Guidelines for Immunosuppressed Patients

These guidelines are intended to minimize the introduction of pathogenic organisms into the gastrointestinal tract by food while maximizing healthy food options for immunosuppressed patients. The guidelines should be coupled with food safety education to assure proper food preparation and storage in the home and hospital kitchen. High risk foods identified as *potential* sources of organisms known to cause infection in immunosuppressed patients are restricted.

In general, autologous transplant patients follow the diet during the first three months after marrow transplant. Allogeneic transplant patients should follow the diet until off all immunosuppressive therapy (ie, cyclosporine, tacrolimus, prednisone).

Food Restrictions
- Raw and undercooked meat (including game), fish, shellfish, poultry, eggs, hot dogs, tofu, sausage, bacon
- Cold smoked fish (salmon) and lox; pickled fish
- Unpasteurized and raw milk and milk products including cheese and yogurt
- Aged cheese (eg, brie, camembert, bleu, roquefort, sharp cheddar, Stilton)
- Refrigerated cheese-based salad dressings (eg, blue cheese), not shelf-stable
- Mexican hot (eg, hot chili pepper) and farmers cheese; feta cheese
- *Unwashed* raw vegetables and fruits and those with visible mold
- Commercial unpasteurized fruit and vegetable juices
- Raw or unpasteurized honey
- All miso products (eg, miso soup); tempeh; maté tea
- Raw, uncooked brewers yeast
- All moldy and out-dated food products
- Unpasteurized beer
- Well water, unless tested yearly and found safe

Source: Clinical Nutrition Department, Fred Hutchinson Cancer Research Center and Nutrition Services Department, Swedish Medical Center, Seattle, Wash. Reprinted with permission.

Monitoring Nutrition Support (5)

Close monitoring of nutrition support is necessary to ensure that the patient's nutrient and fluid needs are met and to minimize PN-associated complications.
- Monitor alterations in medical condition and nutritional status, treatment-related symptoms, and biochemical indices; modify fluid volume, PN substrate, and electrolyte additives, as indicated
- Monitor daily weight and total intake and output volumes during early post-transplant period
- Assess daily oral and intravenous calorie and protein intake levels
- Assess oral and gastrointestinal tolerance to oral feedings

Nutritional Considerations During Marrow Transplantation

Oral and Gastrointestinal Complications

See Box 9.2 for a description of dietary management of common post-transplant nutrition problems (15).

Box 9.2   Dietary Management of Common Nutrition Problems Post-Transplant

Nausea and vomiting
High carbohydrate foods and fluids (crackers, toast, gelatin); non-acidic juices
Small, frequent feedings
Cold, clear liquids and solids
Avoid overly sweet or high fat foods.

Dysgeusia (taste alterations)
Flavored poultry, fish, eggs, dairy products
Herbs, spices, flavor extracts, and marinades may enhance food taste.
Cold, non-odorous foods
Fruit-flavored beverages
Highly aromatic foods
Good oral hygiene
Xerostomia (oral dryness)
Moist foods (stews, casseroles, canned fruit) and liquids
Add extra sauces, gravies, margarine, butter, and broth to foods.
Encourage liquids with meals.
Adding vinegar and pickles to foods may help lessen xerostomia.
Sucking lemon-flavored, sugarless candy may stimulate saliva.
Good oral hygiene
Commercial saline spray may help.

Thick, viscous saliva and mucous
Adequate fluid intake
Clear liquids (tea, popsicles, slushes)
Good oral hygiene

Anorexia
Small, frequent meals of foods high in calories and protein
Use carbohydrate supplements and protein powders.
Create a pleasant mealtime atmosphere with enhancing food aromas, colorful place settings, varied color and textures of foods, and soft music.
Encourage patient participation in grocery shopping and meal planning.
Relaxation techniques and light exercise before meals may help improve food intake.

Oral and esophageal mucositis (inflammation of the mucous membranes of the oral mucosa and esophagus)
Soft- or puree-textured diet
Smooth, bland, moist foods (custard, cream soups, mashed potatoes)
Soft, non-irritating, cold foods (popsicles, ice cream, frozen yogurt, slushes)
Liquid diets
Good oral hygiene

Diarrhea
Low fat, low fiber diet
Avoid caffeine and alcohol.
Cold or room-temperature foods and beverages may be better tolerated.
Low lactose intake
Pancreatic enzyme replacement or lactase enzyme replacement may help.
Encourage adequate fluids to prevent dehydration.

Hepatic Veno-Occlusive Disease (VOD)

Clinical characteristics of VOD (characterized by a fibrous obstruction of the hepatic venules) include: elevated bilirubin, weight gain with concomitant ascites, jaundice, hepatomegaly, and in severe cases, encephalopathy (16). Nutrition management of VOD (4):

- Concentration of PN fluids with reduction of sodium additives to minimize fluid retention
- Monitor lipid utilization; measure lipid clearance if bilirubin increased to >10 mg/dL.
- Remove copper and manganese from PN with persistent hyperbilirubinemia (bilirubin >15 mg/dL).
- With mental status changes, obtain plasma amino acid profile; if aromatic amino acids are twice normal, recommend trial of hepatic failure amino acid solution.

Renal Complications (4)

- Acute renal failure: maximize nutrition support within fluid allowance; correct electrolyte imbalances
- Modify protein intake to 1.25 × recommended dietary allowance.
- Monitor lipid utilization by nephelometric techniques.
- Dialysis: modify vitamin supplementation; provide B-complex with C and folic acid without fat-soluble vitamins.

Graft-versus-Host Disease

Graft-versus-host disease (GVHD) is a T-cell mediated immunologic reaction of engrafted lymphoid cells against the host tissues. The major target organs affected are the skin, liver, and intestinal tract. Therapeutic measures used to prevent or treat GVHD often include multi-drug immunosuppressive agents, many of which have nutritional implications (Table 9.3) (15).

Clinical manifestations of gastrointestinal GVHD include nausea, vomiting, severe abdominal pain and cramping, voluminous watery, green diarrhea, and intestinal bleeding (17). Malabsorption and intestinal protein losses are also characteristic of the mucosal degeneration associated with intestinal GVHD (15). In addition to immunosuppressive drug therapy, a specialized five-phase dietary regimen should be instituted (Table 9.4) (18).

Table 9.3   Mechanisms and Nutritional Implications of GVHD Therapy Medications

Medication (GVHD Prophylaxis/Treatment)	Classification	Mechanism of Action	Nutritional Implications
Anti-thymocyte globulin (ATG)	Immunosuppressant	May eliminate antigen-reactive T-cells (T-lymphocytes) in peripheral blood and/or alteration of T-cell function	Must infuse with normal saline over 8–10 hours, thus may interfere with parenteral nutrition support; may cause nausea, vomiting, diarrhea, and stomatitis
Azathioprine (Imuran®) (GlaxoWellcome, Triangle Park, NJ)	Immunosuppressant	Suppresses hypersensitivities of the cell-mediated type and causes variable alterations in antibody production	Nausea and vomiting; anorexia, and diarrhea when drug is given in large doses; mucosal ulceration, esophagitis, steatorrhea
Beclomethasone dipropionate	Synthetic glucocorticoid	Produces anti-inflammatory and vasoconstrictor effects	Xerostomia; dysgeusia; adrenal insufficiency; nausea
Corticosteroids (Methylprednisolone) (Prednisone) (Dexamethasone)	Synthetic glucocorticoid	Produces anti-inflammatory effects	Sodium and fluid retention resulting in weight gain or hypertension; hyperphagia;; hypokalemia; skeletal muscle catabolism and atrophy, necessitating increased protein requirements; gastric irritation and peptic ulceration; osteoporosis; growth retardation in children; decreased insulin sensitivity and impaired glucose tolerance, resulting in hyperglycemia or steroid-induced diabetes; hypertriglyceridemia
Cyclosporine	Immunosuppressant	Prevents or ameliorates GVHD by suppressing T-cell function	Nausea and vomiting; renal insufficiency, magnesium wasting, potassium wasting
Tacrolimus (Prograf®) (Fujisawa USA, Deerfield, Ill.)	Macrolide immunosuppressant	Suppresses cell-mediated and humoral immune responses	Nephrotoxicity; hyperglycemia; hyperkalemia; hypomagnesemia
Methotrexate	Antimetabolite	Interferes with DNA synthesis by antagonizing folic acid; given intravenously for GVHD prophylaxis and intrathecally for the prevention of central nervous system relapse	Nausea and vomiting mild to moderate; anorexia, mucositis and esophagitis (severe); diarrhea, renal and hepatic implications; decreased absorption of vitamin B_{12}, fat and D-xylose; hepatic fibrosis; change in taste acuity
Mycophenolate mofetil	Immunosuppressant	Enhances availability of mycophenolic acid which inhibits recruitment of leukocytes	Vomiting and diarrhea
PUVA/Psoralen	Photosensitizer	Used in treatment of skin GVHD; modulates immune system, ie,, number and function of circulating lymphocytes, monocytes and macrophages	Nausea, hepatotoxicity
Sirolumus (Rapamune®) (Investigational) (Wyeth-Ayerst Laboratories, St. David's, Penn.)	Immunosuppressant	Inhibits T-cell proliferation	Weight loss; hyperglycemia; anorexia; hypertriglyceridemia
Thalidomide (Investigational)	Glutamic acid derivative	Alters T-cell function	Constipation, nausea, xerostomia
Ursodeoxycholic acid (Actigall®) (Summit Pharmaceuticals, Fort Lee, NJ)	Bile acid	Used in treatment of liver GVHD; displaces retained toxic bile acids in cholestatic or inflammatory hepatic diseases	Nausea and vomiting; diarrhea, dyspepsia

Adapted with permission from Charuhas (15).

Table 9.4   Gastrointestinal GVHD Diet Progression

Phase	Clinical Symptoms	Diet	Clinical Symptoms of Diet Intolerance
1. Bowel rest	GI cramping Large volume watery diarrhea Depressed serum albumin Severely reduced transit time Small bowel obstruction or diminished bowel sounds Nausea and vomiting	Oral: NPO IV: stress energy and protein requirements	
2. Introduction of oral feeding	Minimal GI cramping Diarrhea less than 500 mL/day Guaiac-negative stools Improved transit time (minimum 1.5 hours) Infrequent nausea and vomiting	Oral: isosmotic, low-residue, low-lactose beverages, initially 60 mL every 2–3 hours, for several days IV: as for Phase 1	Increased stool volume or diarrhea Increased emesis Increased abdominal cramping
3. Introduction of solids	Minimal or no GI cramping Formed stool	Oral: allow introduction of solid food, once every 3–4 hours: minimal lactose[a], low fiber, low fat (20-40 g/day)[b], low total acidity, no gastric irritants IV: as for Phase 1	As in Phase 2
4. Expansion of diet	Minimal or no GI cramping Formed stool	Oral: minimal lactose[a], low fiber, low total acidity, no gastric irritants; if stools indicate fat malabsorption: low fat[b] IV: as needed to meet nutritional requirements	As in Phase 2
5. Resumption of regular diet	No GI cramping Normal stool Normal transit time Normal albumin	Oral: progress to regular diet by introducing one restricted food per day: acid foods with meals, fiber-containing foods, lactose-containing foods. Order of addition will vary, depending on individual tolerances and preferences. Patients no longer exhibiting steatorrhea should have the fat restriction liberalized slowly IV: discontinue when oral nutritional intake meets estimated needs	As in Phase 2

[a]Lactose is one of the last disaccharidases to return following villous atrophy. A commercially-prepared lactose solution (Lactaid®) is used to reduce the lactose content of milk by >90%. Lactaid® milk (100% lactose-free) is also commercially available.
[b]Additional calories may be provided by commercially available medium chain triglycerides which do not exacerbate symptoms.
Adapted with permission from Darbinian (18).

Long-term Complications and Management
Chronic Graft-versus-Host Disease

Chronic GVHD develops after day 80 post-transplant with increased frequency in non-identical related and unrelated donors. Nutrition problems reported at one year post-transplant in patients with chronic GVHD include weight gain, weight loss, oral sensitivity, xerostomia, stomatitis, anorexia, reflux symptoms, and diarrhea (19). Community-based nutrition monitoring is necessary following discharge home from transplant centers (19).

Pediatric Issues

Growth and development problems (ie, decreased growth velocity, growth hormone deficiency, and delayed onset of puberty) are frequent in the pediatric population (20). Regular evaluations are necessary to detect occurrence of endocrine dysfunction.

Summary

Marrow transplantation is an intense therapy for malignant and nonmalignant disorders of the bone marrow. It is associated with multiple nutritional challenges, high morbidity and long-term health problems. Dietetic professionals working with this population should be aware of the nutrition-related concerns and need for regular, ongoing nutrition monitoring.

References

1. Charuhas PM. Nutritional Management of the Bone Marrow Transplant Patient. In: Skipper A, ed. *The Dietitian's Handbook of Enteral and Parenteral Nutrition* 2nd ed. Gaithersburg, Md: Aspen Publishing, Inc; 1998:273-294.
2. Secola R. Pediatric blood cell transplantation. *Semin Oncol Nurs.* 1997;13:184-193.
3. Kelly P, Kurtzberg J, Vichinsky E, Lubin B. Umbilical cord blood stem cells: application for the treatment of patients with hemoglobinopathies. *J Pediatr.* 1997;130:695-703.
4. Fred Hutchinson Cancer Research Center, Swedish Medical Center, Veterans Administration Medical Center. *BMT/PBSCT Nutrition Care Criteria.* Seattle, Wash: Fred Hutchinson Cancer Research Center; 1995.
5. Charuhas PM. Pediatric bone marrow transplantation. In: *The American Society for Parenteral and Enteral Nutrition Support Practice Manual.* Silver Spring, Md: A.S.P.E.N; 1998:30-1–30-10.
6. Renal Dietitians Dietetic Practice Group Adjustment in body weight for obese patients (Appendix 8). In: *Suggested Guidelines for Nutrition Care of Renal Patients.* Chicago, Ill: The American Dietetic Association, 1990:34.
7. Geibig CB, Owens JP, Mirtallo JM, Bowers D, Nahikian-Nelms M, Tutschka P. Parenteral nutrition for marrow transplant recipients: evaluation of an increased nitrogen dose. *JPEN.* 1991;15:184-188.
8. Harris JA, Benedict FG. *Biometric Studies of Basal Metabolism in Man.* Washington, DC: Carnegie Institution of Washington; 1919. Publication 279.
9. Altman PL, Dittmer DS, eds. *Metabolism.* Bethesda, Md: Federation of American Societies for Experimental Biology; 1968.
10. Barone MA, ed. The Harriet Lane Handbook. 14th ed. The Johns Hopkins Hospital. St. Louis, Mo: Mosby; 1996.
11. American Medical Association. Department of Foods and Nutrition. Multivitamin preparations for parenteral use. A statement by the nutrition advisory group. *JPEN.* 1979;3:258-262.
12. Cunningham BA. Parenteral Management. In: Lenssen P, Aker SN, eds. *Nutritional Assessment and Management During Marrow Transplantation. A Resource Manual.* Seattle, Wash: Fred Hutchinson Cancer Research Center; 1985:45-61.
13. American Medical Association. Guidelines for essential trace element preparations for parenteral use. A statement by the nutrition advisory group. *JPEN.* 1979;3:263-267.
14. American Academy of Pediatrics. Committee on Nutrition. Commentary on Parenteral Nutrition. *Pediatrics.* 1983;71:547-552.
15. Charuhas PM. Introduction to marrow transplantation. *Oncology Nutrition Dietetic Practice Group Newsletter.* 1994;2:2-9.
16. Baglin TP. Veno-occlusive disease of the liver complicating bone marrow transplantation. *Bone Marrow Transplant.* 1994;13:1-4.
17. McDonald GB, Shulman HM, Sullivan KM, Spencer GD. Intestinal and hepatic complications of human bone marrow transplantation. Part I. *Gastroenterology.* 1986;90:460-477.

18. Darbinian J, Schubert MM. Special Management Problems. In: Lenssen P, Aker SN, eds. *Nutritional Assessment and Management During Marrow Transplantation. A Resource Manual.* Seattle, Wash: Fred Hutchinson Cancer Research Center; 1985:63–80.

19. Lenssen P, Sherry ME, Cheney CL, Nims JW, Sullivan KM, Stern JM, Moe G, Aker SN. Prevalence of nutrition-related problems among long-term survivors of allogeneic marrow transplantation. *J Am Diet Assoc.* 1990;90:835–842.

20. Sanders JE. Bone marrow transplantation for pediatric malignancies. *Pediatr Clin North Am.* 1997;44:1005–1020.

10

Medical Nutrition Therapy in Pediatric Oncology

Ruth Williams, MS, RD   Karen Smith, MS, RD, CNSD

Malnutrition is not common in children with newly diagnosed neoplastic diseases. However, certain conditions, diagnoses, and therapies can lead to malnutrition. Causes of malnutrition in children with cancer may be secondary to the cancer itself or to the treatment. Disease may cause anorexia, early satiety, weight loss, growth failure, and weakness (1). Additionally, treatments such as radiation and chemotherapy cause significant negative side effects on nutrition status (ie, nausea, vomiting, diarrhea, mucositis, decreased saliva production, altered taste perception) (1).

Radiation therapy may be the primary treatment modality when a tumor is either unresectable or radiosensitive. Radiation also is used in combination with chemotherapy and/or surgery. A consequence of radiation therapy is obligatory damage to healthy tissue within the irradiated field. Symptoms of this damage (ie, altered bone growth in irradiated areas, problems with cognition and learning, hearing loss) may not develop for up to 10 years (1).

There are numerous nutritional consequences associated with chemotherapeutic agents. Side effects produced depend upon the type of drug, dosage given, duration of treatment, rates of excretion, and individual susceptibility. See Chapter 6, *Chemotherapy and Nutrition Implications,* for a list of common chemotherapeutic drugs used and their side effects (1).

In addition to problems associated with disease and therapy, practitioners must also consider the growth and development needs of children. Although in adults with cancer, practitioners may strive to maintain weight, this is not necessarily appropriate in children. Careful monitoring of height and weight to achieve adequate growth is more appropriate in children. Although some therapy may cause temporary growth stunting (ie, bone marrow transplant) this should not be a long-term side effect. Adequate calories and protein should be provided so the child will continue to grow as normally as possible.

Another consideration in caring for the child with cancer is the parents. Parents frequently are anxious and usually very concerned about their child's intake. Often, they place additional stress on the child to eat and may need assurance that due to his/her medical condition, the child is unable to eat at that time. Assurance that the health care team is monitoring the child's nutrition status and will provide support when needed can help to alleviate some of the parents' concerns.

Nutrition intervention in children with cancer is an important adjunct to increasingly complex oncologic therapy. Nutrition therapy for the prevention or reversal of protein energy malnutrition is especially important in children who cannot afford to lose weight. Development of an institution-specific risk protocol should assist in focusing nutrition therapy on high risk populations. Table 10.1 shows how one pediatric oncology center (St. Jude Children's Research Hospital in Memphis, Tennessee) developed a risk stratification protocol for nutrition screening and assessment.

Table 10.1   Risk Stratification Protocol for Nutrition Screening and Assessment

Level	Conditions	Assessment/Care Plan	Reassessment
1	a. Nutrition support (enteral, parenteral) b. Bone marrow transplant—initial c. Weight loss (3%–5% in past month) d. NPO >3 days	24 hours	Minimum 2 times per week
2	a. Non-chemotherapy induced nausea/ vomiting, diarrhea b. Mucositis/oral problems c. Modified diet	72 hours	Minimum 1 time a week
3	a. Newly diagnosed treatment on protocols known to result in nutrition problems based on chemotherapy used, diagnosis, location of disease (ie, head/neck/brain tumor) and age 3 years	72 hours	As indicated

Source: Department of Clinical Nutrition, St. Jude Children's Research Hospital, Memphis, Tenn. Used with permission.

Assessment

The following are recommendations for determining patients at nutrition risk.

A. Identification of Malnourished and/or Problem Patients
    1. Risk factors
        a. Weight/height
            (1) 90% of ideal body weight (IBW) or usual body weight (mild) (See section B for description of ideal body weight.)
            (2) 85% of IBW or usual body weight (moderate)
            (3) 80% of IBW or usual body weight (severe).
        b. Weight loss of >5% over 1-month period or less.
        c. Albumin <3.2 g/dL.
        d. Impending therapy will diminish nutrition status.
        e. Less than 50% of required oral intake for 3 days.

    2. Patients identified as "at risk" will be divided into categories:
        a. 1st degree: low risk (nourished); 0–1 risk factors
        b. 2nd degree: moderate risk (potential for malnutrition); 2–3 risk factors
        c. 3rd degree: high risk (malnourished); 3+ risk factors

All "at risk" patients should receive an in-depth nutrition assessment which may include but not be limited to:
• biochemical assessment of nutritional status based on available laboratory data (albumin, pre-albumin, BUN, creatinine)
• in-depth diet, appetite and nutritional history (note physical and psychological difficulties related to eating)
• estimation of any nutrient deficiencies, nutrient needs, and IBW
• food/drug interactions
• food intolerance or allergies
• conditions that may affect gastrointestinal system (ingestion, absorption)
• food preferences based on personal tastes, culture, religion
• present diet prescription
• recommended rationale and goals of therapy; therapeutic plan; patient monitoring
• any information given by other disciplines (e.g., social work, pastoral care, psychology, occupational, and physical therapy) that is pertinent to nutrition and is to be incorporated into the nutrition care plan. Such information may be obtained through other disciplines at team rounds, in progress notes, or by discussions with other health care team members.

B. Calculation of Ideal Body Weight (IBW)
  1. Normal weight patient
     a. Plot height on weight/height side of National Center for Health Statistics (NCHS) growth charts (4).
     b. Plot weight at 50th percentile for height.
     c. This is IBW.
  2. Ideal body weight in patients with amputations (5)
     a. Calculate ideal body weight by the above method.
     b. Determine percent weight of the amputated body segment using following table:
        Estimation of body segmented weights:

Entire upper limb:	6.5%
Forearm and hand:	2.3%
Hand:	0.8%
Entire lower limb:	18.5%
Above-knee amputation:	7.1%
Below-knee amputation:	5.9%
Foot amputation:	1.8%

     c. Take current weight, without the prosthesis, and add the weight of the amputated limb:
        Current weight X (100% + % weight of limb expressed as a decimal) = adjusted weight.
        Use this adjusted weight to compare patients' weight with ideal weight.
  3. Adjusted body weight for patients >120% IBW:
     Adjusted BW ([actual weight – IBW] X .25) + ideal weight
     Use this adjusted BW as ideal weight (6).

Determination of Energy, Protein, and Fat Requirements for the Pediatric/Adolescent Oncology Patient

Calorie and Protein Requirements

Recommendations for protein intake in infants and children assume an adequate caloric intake. The RDA does not make allowances for any disease state, nor does it include catch-up growth and stress. At least 30 calories should be provided for every gram of protein delivered, to meet basal needs. Protein calories are not to be used as part of calorie requirements (7). For children who have normal visceral protein stores, no stressful therapy impending, and no need for accelerated growth or repletion, use RDA based on age. For patients with greater requirements due to stress, monitor visceral protein (ie, albumin, prealbumin) and adjust protein as needed (typically 1.5–2.0 times the RDA). See Tables 10.2 and 10.3.

Table 10.2   RDA Table for Calories (7)

	Age (years)	Calories per kg
Infants	0.0–0.5	108
	0.1–1.0	98
Children	1–3	102
	4–6	90
	7–10	70
Males	11–14	55
	15–18	45
Females	11–14	47
	15–18	40

Table 10.3   RDA Table for Proteins (7)

	Age (years)	Protein (g/kg)
Infants	0.05–0.5	2.2
	0.5–1.0	1.6
Children	1–3	1.2
	4–6	1.1
	7–10	1.0
Males	11–14	1.0
	15–18	0.9
Females	11–14	1.0
	15–18	0.8

Failure to Thrive (FTT)

In the patient with FTT, catch-up growth is desirable. Catch-up growth refers to growth occurring at a rate greater than expected for age and sex. The patient's ability to "catch up" is dependent on how many calories the patient is able to consume. The timing, severity, nature, and duration of the nutritional insult may directly impact potential for catch-up growth (8).

Children are considered FTT if they meet one of the following criteria:

a. Weight/height below 5th percentile
b. Weight or height deficit of more than 2 percentiles
c. Less than 80% of ideal body weight based on height

Caloric requirements of the FTT child (8):

$$\frac{Kcal}{kg} = \frac{\text{RDA for age kcal} \times \text{IBW} \left(\frac{wt}{ht} \text{ at 50th percentile}\right)}{\text{actual weight (kg)}}$$

Protein requirements of the FTT child (8):

$$Pro(g) = \frac{\text{Protein required for weight age (g/kg/day)} \times \text{IBW (kg)}}{\text{actual weight (kg)}}$$

Fat Requirements

Fat supplies 40% to 50% of the energy consumed in infancy and about 40% of the energy consumed after infancy by individuals in developed countries. For healthy children over 2 years of age, a diet is recommended that meets the American Academy of Pediatrics (AAP) and National Cholesterol Education Program (NCEP) (24) of <30% total calories from fat, <10% total calories from saturated fatty acids, and a serum value of <300 mg/dL cholesterol. Studies have shown that adequate growth can be achieved with such a diet (9,10,11,12). The primary goal in determining a child's diet should be adequate growth and development. Infants and toddlers under 2 years of age should not have a fat or cholesterol restricted diet. Fat at this age is necessary for development and as a source of energy. Because of caloric density, fat can be very important in lean and physically active children, children with small appetites, and children able to eat only small volumes of food at one time (11). For those children, it may be necessary to exceed NCEP recommendations. Fat is protein-sparing, because its availability reduces the body's need to use protein as an energy source. Fats are sources of and facilitate the absorption of the fat-soluble vitamins A, D, E, and K.

1. RDA
   a. RDA for fat has not been established.
   b. The diets of infants and toddlers under age 2 should not be restricted to less than 30% total calories from fat and cholesterol. In infants, 30%–55% of calories from fat is appropriate (11).
   c. Individuals over 2 years of age may have a diet of less than 30% total calories from fat without compromising growth and development (13,14). More than 50% of calories from fat is not recommended.
2. Essential Fatty Acids
   Essential fatty acids (EFA) are precursors of the phospholipids in cell membranes and of prostaglandins, thromboxanes, and leukotrienes.
   a. Polyunsaturated linoleic acid is considered an essential fatty acid. The minimal requirements for linoleic acid are 2% to 4% of total calories required (25–100 mg/kg/day) or 8% to 10% of estimated calories from fat (13). Other sources suggest that 1% to 2% of dietary calories as linoleic acid will prevent EFA deficiency. For example, a child eating 1,200 calories would require 1.3 g to 2.6 g linoleic acid/day. Infants consuming 100 kcal/kg body weight per day require 0.2 g linoleic acid per kilogram. Adults require 3 g to 6 g per day (13).

b. Patients on long-term TPN may require lipids in order to avoid EFA deficiency if they are not eating sufficient fat. Signs and symptoms of EFA deficiency include dry, flaky skin, possibly as eczema, with inflammation of the skin and dry, scaly lesions. Other symptoms include dry hair, poor growth, decreased platelets, and impaired wound healing. Children on TPN should not go without fat for more than 3 weeks. If unable to give intravenous (IV) fat, an estimate of fat taken by mouth must be assessed and counseling provided to take in adequate amounts (15).

c. Fat supplied in TPN should be 20% to 60% of calories (15).

d. In infants, begin at 1 g/kg/day of fat and advance by 0.5 to 1.0 g/kg/day to goal. Upper limit is 4 g/kg/day (15).

e. In children and teenagers, begin at 1 g/kg/day and increase by 1 g/kg/day to goal. Upper limit is 2.5 to 3 g/kg/day (15).

Route of Nutrition Support

Methods for preventing or treating nutrition depletion in this patient population vary, ranging from counseling for encouragement of high-quality oral intake to aggressive intervention via parenteral or enteral access. Often the side effects and toxicities of treatment result in the patient not being able to consume adequate oral intake. At this point, alternate routes of nutrition support should be considered. A multidisciplinary team approach is optimal in order to integrate nutrition planning into the oncology treatment scheme. In addition, effective nutrition strategies will depend on the support and involvement of the family. A comprehensive care plan that includes nutrition and addresses the needs of the whole child is likely to be successful. Institution-specific criteria regarding the route of support and appropriate time for intervention is recommended. Figure 10.1 is an example of the decision-making algorithm for nutrition support at St. Jude Children's Research Hospital in Memphis, Tennessee.

Oral Support

Every attempt should be made to encourage food intake via normal eating. Foods can be altered to make them higher in calories, softer, or higher in protein, depending on the child's specific needs. See Appendix A for general information on symptom management.

Enteral Support

Enteral support should be the first choice of nutrition therapy for individuals with intact, functioning gastrointestinal tracts. Mathew et al, conducted a retrospective review of 33 children with malignancies who received nutrition support by gastrostomy tube (13). Their study objective was twofold, to assess the nature and frequency of complications and their relation to the type of gastrostomy feeding device, and to evaluate the effectiveness of nutrition support by gastrostomy feeding. Although most patients (64%) had a minor complication (ie, reaction to insertion site), 82% of the patients in this study were able to maintain or achieve ideal body weight. They concluded that gastrostomy tube feeding was associated with minor complications, and that this form of nutrition therapy permitted effective nutrition support.

Figure 10.1   Algorithm for Nutrition Support

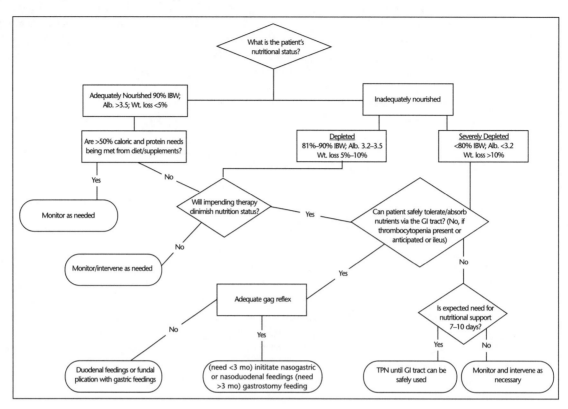

©1997, The Clinical Nutrition Service's Standards of Care, St. Jude Children's Research Hospital, Memphis, Tenn. Used with permission.

Parenteral Support

Parenteral nutrition should only be utilized when the gastrointestinal tract cannot be used due to surgery, persistent vomiting, intractable diarrhea, graft-versus-host disease of the gut, ileus, obstruction, or radiation requiring NPO status for a prolonged period (14). Institution-specific criteria regarding route of support and appropriate time for intervention are required (Figure 10.1).

References

1. Sheard NF, Clark NG. Nutrition management of pediatric oncology patients. In: Baker SB, Baker RD, Davis A, eds. *Pediatric Enteral Nutrition*. New York: Chapman and Hall; 1994:387–398.
2. *Standards of Care*. St. Jude Children's Research Hospital, Memphis, Tennessee. Unpublished manuscript.
3. Hamil PVV, Drizd TA, Johnson CL, Reed RB, Roche AF, Moore WM. Physical growth: National Center for Health Statistics percentiles. *AM J Clin Nutr*. 1979:32:607–629. Data from the National Center for Health Statistics (NCHS), Hyattsville, Md.
4. Osterkamplk: current perspective on assessment of human body proportions of relevance to amputees. *JAM Diet Assoc* 1995;95(2):215–218.
5. Lysen LK. *Quick Reference to Clinical Dietetics*. Gaithersburg, Md:ASPEN; 1997.
6. Wilkens K (ed). Suggested guidelines for Nutrition care of renal patients. Chicago, Ill:American Dietetic Association, 1986; 34.

7. National Research Council, National Academy of Sciences. *Recommended Dietary Allowances.* 9th ed. Washington, DC: National Academy of Sciences Press; 1989.

8. Cox JH, Cooning SW. Parenteral Nutrition. In: Oueen PM, Long CE, eds. *Handbook of Pediatric Nutrition.* Gaitherburg, Md: ASPEN; 1993: 279-314.

9. American Academy of Pediatrics committed on cholesterol. statement on Cholesterol. *Pediatrics.* 1992;90:469-473.

10. Kleinman RE, Finberg LF, Klish WJ, Laver RM. Dietary guidelines for children. *J Nutr.* 1996;126:1028S-1030S.

11. NCEP Expert Panel on Blood cholesterol levels in children and adolescents. National Cholesterol Education program (NCEP). *Pediatures.* 1992:89:525-527.

12. Shea S, Basch CE, Stein AD, Contento IL, Irigoyen M, Zybert P. Is there a relationship between dietary fat and stature or growth in children three to five years of age. *Pediatrics.* 1993;92(4):579-586.

13. Hardy SC, Kleinman RE. Fat and cholesterol in the diet of infants and young children: implications for growth, development, and long-term health. *J Pediatrics.* 125:569-77.

14 Sigman-Grant M, Zimmerman S, Kirs-Etherton PM. Dietary approaches for reducing fat intake of pre-school age children. *Pediatrics.* 1994;91:955-960.

15. Skipper A, Marian M. Parenteral nutrition. In: *Nutrition Support Dietetics Core Curriculum*, 2nd ed. Silver Spring, Md: ASPEN, 1993: 105-123.

16. Mathew P, Bowman L, Williams R. Complications and effectiveness of gastrostomy feeds in pediatric cancer patients. *J Pediatric Hematol Oncol.* 1996;18(1):81-85.

17. Bowman L, Williams R, Sanders M, Smith K, et al. Algorithm for nutritional support. *Int J Cancer.* 1998;11(supplement):76-80.

11

Enteral Nutrition in Adult Medical/Surgical Oncology

Renee Piazza-Barnett, MEd, RD, CNSD   Laura E. Matarese, MS, RD, FADA, CNSD

Cancer-related malnutrition has been associated with increased morbidity and mortality and decreased response to therapy (1,2). The cause of malnutrition is multifactorial, resulting from diminished intake, increased requirements, and metabolic alterations. Malnourished cancer patients may benefit from nutrition support in an attempt to reverse or, at least, lessen the progression of malnutrition. Patients with active disease who are receiving treatment should receive nutrition support if they are unable to consume adequate nutrition. Although provision of nutrition has been shown to increase tumor growth, this was in an experimental animal model with large tumor burden (3). Human tumor burdens are smaller and provision of adequate nutrition may enhance response to anticancer therapy (2). If the gastrointestinal (GI) tract is functional, accessible, and safe to use, enteral nutrition, either by oral supplementation or tube feedings, is the preferred method of nutrition support in the medical/surgical oncology patient.

Benefits of Enteral Feeding

Physiological

Nutrients are absorbed by the portal system with subsequent delivery to the liver, which supports visceral protein synthesis and regulation of metabolic processes.

Bacterial translocation, which is the passage of enteric flora and/or endotoxins through the epithelial mucosa to the portal circulation and mesenteric lymph nodes, is prevented. The translocation of intestinal bacteria and endotoxins into systemic circulation may lead to sepsis and multiple system organ failure in the cancer patient (1,4,5–13). Animal studies have demonstrated that even short periods of total parenteral nutrition (TPN) are associated with mucosal atrophy and the associated translocation of bacteria, which is reversed by enteral nutrition (4,14–21).

Certain amino acids, such as glutamine, which may be conditionally essential during periods of stress, are provided (22). Glutamine is in enteral formulas as intact protein, short-chain peptides, or free amino acids. Inadequate levels of glutamine have been postulated to be associated with intestinal atrophy and decreased numbers of IgA-producing lymphocytes (23–29). Commercially available parenteral amino acid solutions do not contain free glutamine because of pharmaceutical considerations during manufacturing. Although glutamine may be unstable in parenteral solutions, it has been used in various research protocols involving TPN (30–40).

Fiber, which is essential to gut function, can be provided. Short-chain fatty acids from colonic fermentation of fiber provide fuel to the cells of the colon (41,42). This results in a nutrient-rich environment in which bacteria proliferate and add solid mass to the stool (43). Soy polysaccharide is the most common fiber additive found in enteral nutrition formulas. It is inexpensive and easily suspended in liquid and has been shown to prevent diarrhea and normalize bowel function (44–47). Fructooligosaccharides (FOS) are short-chain simple sugars linked together by indigestible bonds, which have been shown to selectively stimulate the growth of beneficial bacteria, resulting in the reduction of pathogenic bacteria (48).

The small bowel continues to function in critically ill patients who are experiencing gastric atony (eg, after a vagotomy for gastric cancer), so feeding into the small bowel can usually be initiated immediately after access is obtained (2,49).

Immunologic secretory proteins are stimulated, and feeding into the gastrointestinal tract helps to blunt the catabolic response (50).

Safety

Although enteral nutrition has its own set of potential complications, it is generally considered safer than parenteral nutrition (see section on complications below). Enteral delivery of nutrients decreases infectious complications in critically injured patients compared with intravenously fed patients (51). Also, it may decrease postoperative complications when given before surgery to malnourished cancer patients (52). Enteral nutrition avoids complications related to central venous catheters (eg, catheter sepsis, pneumothorax, catheter embolism, arterial laceration, and hydrothorax) in a group of patients who are often immunosuppressed and at high risk for infectious complications.

Economic

Formula, equipment, and personnel is less costly for enteral nutrition than for TPN (53,54).

Indications for Enteral Nutrition

Enteral nutrition is indicated when the gastrointestinal tract is functional, yet oral nutrient intake is insufficient to meet needs. The American Dietetic Association (ADA) has identified important specific indicators to monitor that may help determine if a patient is a candidate for nutrition support (55). These are:

1. Patient is NPO or on a clear liquid diet without nutrition support for 5 days.
2. Patient is at moderate or high risk as identified by screening and assessment (assessment tools include the scored Patient-Generated Subjective Global Assessment, institution-specific guidelines, and the Oncology Screening Tool) (2).
3. Moderate or high-risk patients/caregivers demonstrate knowledge/skills required to implement nutrition care plan for discharge.

Specific Indications for Enteral Nutrition (1)

- **Head and neck cancer** Patients with advanced head and neck cancer suffer from malnutrition due to the malignancy itself, often with an associated history of chronic alcohol abuse. In addition, treatment of head and neck cancer (eg, radiation, surgery) significantly contributes to the severe malnutrition seen in these patients.

  Head and neck cancer patients may be fed enterally, either by small-bore nasogastric tubes or percutaneously-placed gastrostomies or jejunostomies (see Table 11.1). If the endoscopic route is not possible, surgical placement of a gastrostomy or jejunostomy tube is an option.

- **Esophageal cancer** The malnutrition associated with esophageal cancer is due in part to mechanical obstruction and anorexia, but tumor-dependent metabolic alterations also contribute to the cachexia syndrome (56). Therapy associated with esophageal cancer (eg, radiation, chemotherapy, surgical treatment) also result in worsening nutritional conditions. Endoscopic or surgical placement of feeding tubes into the stomach or duodenum is frequently successful in feeding this group of patients (Table 11.1).

- **Pancreatic cancer** Pancreatic cancer is associated with a high incidence of malnutrition and weight loss (1). There are four main reasons for this: 1) gastric outlet obstruction from the tumor, 2) fat malabsorption and vitamin K deficiency due to biliary obstruction, 3) malabsorption secondary to pancreatic insufficiency, 4) early satiety and delayed emptying as a result of gastric resection. Enteral nutrition in this group of patients may be administered through a jejunostomy tube (Table 11.1). Also, pancreatic enzyme replacement and medium chain triglycerides may be indicated if a total pancreatectomy is performed.

- **Gastric cancer** Gastric resection for gastric cancer could cause rapid transit, dumping syndrome and hypoglycemia, and possible deficiences of iron, calcium, vitamin B12, and fat-soluble vitamins (1). Percutaneous or surgical placement of feeding tubes into the jejunum may be used to feed this group of patients. Elemental or predigested enteral formulas may be considered if malabsorption is suspected.

- **Chemotherapy** Nausea, vomiting, mucositis, and GI dysfunction due to chemotherapeutic agents may worsen existing malnutrition in the cancer patient. Also, increased toxicity from chemotherapy is associated with poor nutritional status in this population (57). At this time, no strong evidence supports enteral nutrition as effective in patients with advanced disease undergoing chemotherapy (1). However, there are a few studies looking at patients with less advanced tumors.

- **Radiation therapy** In addition to chemotherapy, radiation therapy contributes to the cancer patient's already-malnourished state. Depending on the area of irradiation, nutritional alterations may result from nausea and vomiting, mucositis, dysphagia, diarrhea, enteritis, and malabsorption. Experimental evidence supports enteral nutrition as a form of prophylaxis against radiation therapy (58). Although similar to the data in chemotherapy trials, studies have not shown that nutritional support during radiotherapy improves tumor response or overall survival (1).

Table 11.1   Enteral Access for Specific Areas of Cancer

Site of Cancer	Enteral Access	Administration
Head and Neck	Nasogastric	Continuous, bolus, or intermittent
	Nasojejunal	Continuous or cycled
	Gastrostomy (percutaneous or surgical)	Continuous, bolus, intermittent, or cycled
	Jejunostomy (percutaneous or surgical)	Continuous or cycled
Esophageal	Gastrostomy (percutaneous or surgical)	Continuous, bolus, intermittent, or cycled
	Jejunostomy (percutaneous or surgical)	Continuous or cycled
Pancreatic	Jejunostomy (percutaneous or surgical)	Continuous or cycled
Gastric	Jejunostomy (percutaneous or surgical)	Continuous or cycled

Contraindications for Enteral Nutrition

There are also conditions in which enteral nutrition may be contraindicated (49). This would include any situation where the gastrointestinal tract is nonfunctional, inaccessible, or when extended bowel rest is required.

- Mechanical obstruction
- Adynamic ileus
- Severe gastrointestinal bleeding
- Severe diarrhea
- Intractable vomiting
- Gastrointestinal fistula
- Severe enterocolitis
- High aspiration risk
- Bowel rest
- Prognosis not consistent with aggressive nutrition

Formula Selection

Selection of formulas is based on several factors. If digestive capability and absorptive capacity are impaired, a predigested formula should be used. The patient's ability to handle fluid volume should also be considered and in some instances, a calorically dense formula may be necessary. Finally, the patient may have a pre-existing medical condition which would necessitate the use of a disease-specific formula. There are many formulas available to provide enteral nutrition (59) and they can be grouped into three main categories: Polymeric, Predigested, and Modular formulas (see Table 11.2).

Table 11.2   Enteral Nutritional Products

Type of Product	Caloric Density	Protein Density	Osmolality	Characteristics
Polymeric				
Standard	1.0 kcal/mL to 1.2 kcal/mL	Moderate	Isotonic or hypertonic	General tube feeding requirements
High Nitrogen	1.0 kcal/mL to 1.5 kcal/mL	High	Isotonic or hypertonic	Indicated for patients with increased protein needs
Fiber Supplemented	1.0 kcal/mL to 1.5 kcal/mL	Moderate or high	Isotonic or hypertonic	Aids in normalizing bowel function
Concentrated	1.5 kcal/mL to 2.0 kcal/mL	Moderate or high	Hypertonic	Indicated for fluid restricted patients
Disease Specific	1.0 kcal/mL to 2.0 kcal/mL	Low, moderate, or high	Isotonic or hypertonic	Indicated for specific disease states (eg, renal/hepatic/respiratory failure, glucose intolerance, stress/trauma)
Predigested	1.0 kcal/mL to 1.5 kcal/mL	Moderate or high (as tri- or di-peptides and/or free amino acids)	Hypertonic	Indicated for patients with impaired digestion or absorption. Generally low in fat and/or provide the fat in the form of MCTs
Modular	Highly variable	Highly variable	Hypotonic or isotonic	Individual carbohydrate, protein, or fat components. Used to supplement oral diets or tube feedings, or design new products

Polymeric

These formulas are nutritionally complete, usually lactose-free, and are casein or soy protein isolate–based. Since nutrients are in an intact molecular form, normal digestion and absorption are required. These formulas supply all necessary nutrients for complete nutrition generally in two liters (60). Polymeric formulas are available in the following varieties:

- **Standard** General tube feeding requirements, 1.0 kcal/mL to 1.2 kcal/mL, moderate in protein content, isotonic or hypertonic
- **High nitrogen** Indicated for patients with increased protein needs, generally supplying 40 gm Pro/L to 66gm Pro/L
- **Fiber supplemented** Aids in normalizing bowel function, the range varies from 1.9 gm to 3.3 gm of total dietary fiber (TDF) per 250 mL of "blenderized" formula and from 2.5 gm to 5.9 gm of TDF per 250 mL of formulas containing soy polysaccharide
- **Concentrated** Indicated for fluid restricted patients, 1.5 kcal/mL to 2.0 kcal/mL
- **Disease-specific** Renal, hepatic, glucose intolerance, pulmonary, stress/trauma

Predigested

These formulas are indicated for patients with impaired digestion and/or absorption, which frequently occur as a complication of chemotherapy, radiation therapy, and after some surgeries (eg, pancreatectomy). Protein is provided as tri-peptides, di-peptides, and/or free amino acids. They are generally low in fat and/or provide the fat in the form of medium chain triglycerides (MCTs). Due to their hydrolyzed nature, predigested formulas are usually hypertonic. They tend to be more expensive than polymeric formulas.

Modular

These products supply a single nutrient or a combination of nutrients and consist primarily of intact macronutrient sources (60). They are used to alter the caloric or protein content of a base formula. An oral diet can be enhanced or a new tube feeding designed through the use of modular formulas. For example, a modular protein supplement can be used to increase the protein content of an enteral product without increasing the caloric density.

Fluid

Most enteral formulas contain from 70 percent to 85 percent water. The majority of patients who are solely supported by tube feeds require additional water to meet hydration requirements (eg, 150 mL water flushes every four hours to six hours). This is especially important in patients receiving high nitrogen or fiber supplemented formulas or who have increased losses due to fevers, diarrhea, chest tubes, fistula, ostomies, or gastric decompression tubes. See Chapter 4, *Calorie, Protein, Fluid, and Micronutrient Requirements*, for specific calculations of fluid requirements.

Types of Enteral Access (49, 61)

There are two types of access through which enteral nutrition can be provided. A nasoenteric tube is used for short-term feeding (less than four weeks) due to low cost and ease of placement (62). A feeding enterostomy is used for permanent or long term nutrition (generally four weeks or longer). See Table 11.3 for a comparison of various enteral access devices.

Table 11.3   Enteral Access Devices

Enteral Device	Aspiration Potential	Dumping Potential	Placement Method	Longevity Potential
Nasogastric	High	Low	Bedside	Short-term
Nasoduodenal	Moderate	Moderate	Bedside Fluoroscopic Endoscopic	Short-term
Nasojejunal	Low	High	Bedside Fluoroscopic Endoscopic	Short-term
Esophago-gastrostomy	High	Low	Surgical	Long-term
Gastrostomy	Moderate	Low	Surgical	Long-term
Jejunostomy	Low	High	Surgical	Long-term
PEG	Moderate	Low	Endoscopic	Long-term
PEJ	Low	High	Endoscopic	Long-term

Nasoenteric Access

- **Nasogastric** Temporary access device of choice in most patients (62). Used in patients with completely functioning gastrointestinal tracts. Not indicated in patients at high risk for aspiration. Endoscopy and/or fluoroscopy not required for placement.
- **Nasoduodenal** Temporary access device. May require endoscopy, fluoroscopy, or prokinetic/gastric motility agents. Used in patients at high risk for aspiration.
- **Nasojejunal** Temporary access device. May require endoscopy, fluoroscopy, or prokinetic agents. Used in patients at high risk for aspiration.

Feeding Enterostomies

- **Open tube gastrostomy** Surgical incision with placement of gastrostomy tube through the abdominal wall.
- **Laparoscopic gastrostomy** For permanent or long-term feedings (63). Done under general anesthesia in conjunction with other laparoscopic procedures. Surgical incision with placement of gastrostomy tube through the abdominal wall.
- **Percutaneous endoscopic gastrostomy (PEG)** Most popular nonoperative procedure for obtaining permanent access (62). Formed by the placement of a tube through a percutaneous hole that passes from the stomach through the anterior abdominal wall. Upper endoscopy is used to assist with placement. May be done on an outpatient basis.
- **Open tube jejunostomy** Surgical placement of a feeding tube through the abdominal wall into the jejunum. Usually placed at least 20 centimeters beyond the ligament of Treitz (64).
- **Percutaneous endoscopic jejunostomy (PEJ)** Permanent jejunal feeding tube placed by way of endoscopy (64). May be placed directly into the jejunum.

- **Laparoscopic jejunostomy** Laparoscopic placement of a feeding tube through the abdominal wall into the jejunum (63). Done under general anesthesia in conjunction with other laparoscopic procedures.
- **Jejunal extension tube (JET)-PEG** Jejunal feeding tube is placed through a PEG tube. Provides jejunal feedings with simultaneous stomach decompression (65).
- **Cervical pharyngostomy** Surgical placement of a feeding tube into the pharynx or cervical esophagus and passed into the stomach. Adjunct to surgery for head and neck tumors or trauma to the maxillofacial region (66).

Administration

The method of administration used to provide enteral nutrition depends on the location of the feeding tube, patient tolerance to the feeding regimen, and overall nutritional goals. Bolus, intermittent, continuous, and cyclic are the four methods of tube feeding administration.

Bolus

Bolusing of tube feeding involves the rapid delivery (20 minutes or less) of 240 mL to 400 mL of formula several times a day. A syringe is used to infuse the feeding into the stomach. This method is more frequently used in home care or with rehabilitation patients to allow them to return to normal activities of daily living (64). Feedings given by this method can sometimes result in nausea, diarrhea, vomiting, distension, cramps, or aspiration. Intolerance to bolus feedings can be managed by changing to an intermittent delivery (see below) or providing continuously via a cycle (see below).

Intermittent

With intermittent feedings, up to 400 mL of formula is delivered over a 20- to 30-minute period several times per day by gravity drip or an infusion pump. Many of the gastrointestinal problems associated with bolus delivery are eliminated, but tolerance may still be poor in some patients. Home care or rehabilitation patients may also use intermittent feedings more frequently than hospitalized patients.

Continuous and Cyclic

Feedings may be delivered continuously via gravity drip or, more often, an infusion pump. They can be delivered over 24 hours or cycled (eg, anywhere from six hours to eight hours during sleep or the more frequent 10 hours to 12 hours), so as to allow the patient mobility when not hooked up to the feeding. These types of feedings are necessary when the tube is in the duodenum or jejunum. Continuous feedings into the stomach may be a prophylaxis against stress ulceration while simultaneously providing nutrition support (64).

Initiation and Advancement

Initiating enteral feeding with isotonic or hypertonic tube feeding formulas instead of hypotonic formulas has been advocated (67). Continuous full-strength tube feedings can be initiated at 20 mL to 50 mL/hour. Progression may range from 10 mL to 20 mL/hour several times daily until the goal rate is achieved (68). Transition to bolus or intermittent is best done after tolerance to continuous feedings is demonstrated.

Complications (61)

Although generally considered to be safer than parenteral nutrition, enteral nutrition is not totally innocuous. Complications related to the delivery of enteral nutrition may be classified into three categories; mechanical, gastrointestinal, and metabolic (see Table 11.4).

Table 11.4   Complications of Enteral Feeding

Complication	Possible Causes	Prevention/Therapy
Displacement/migration	Coughing, vomiting, uncooperative patient	Replace tube and confirm placement.
Obstruction	Crushed medications	Thoroughly crush medications; use liquid medications.
	Incompletely dissolved formula	Mix formulas thoroughly.
	Failure to irrigate	Adequate flushing
High residuals	Decreased gastric motility	Elevate HOB 30°. Gastric stimulants Check residuals frequently. Small bowel feedings
Aspiration; gastric retention, gastric reflux	Altered gastric motility or gag reflux Patient flat in bed Displaced tube	Continuous infusion Check residual. Elevate HOB 30°. Monitor tube placement. Position tube distal to ligament of Treitz.
Nausea/vomiting Cramping Distension Bloating Hypermotility	Formula administration Lactose intolerance Antibiotic therapy Cold formula	Advance rate and concentration gradually. Use lactose-free formulas. Administer at room temperature.
Diarrhea	Formula administration	Advance rate and concentration gradually; continuous infusion; decrease rate and/or concentration temporarily.
	Overfeeding	Reduce excessive calorie intake.
	Lactose intolerance	Lactose-free formula
	Malnutrition (hypoalbuminemia)	Use elemental diet initially; administer albumin.
	Malabsorption	Pancreatic enzymes
	Bacterial contamination	Change solutions frequently. Clean technique
Constipation	Inadequate fluid Decreased gastric motility Inadequate bulk Medications Inactivity	Increase free water. Stool softener Increase fiber. Prune juice Increase activity.

Mechanical

Feeding tube displacement and migration is a serious complication and may result in feedings being delivered to a location other than the one intended. This can result in aspiration, diarrhea, or peritonitis (with gastrostomy or jejunostomy tubes). Verification of tube placement by x-ray should be done before feedings are started or anytime tube malpositioning is suspected.

Feeding tube obstruction may occur due to formula coagulation, obstruction by pill fragments, tube kinking, and precipitation by incompatible medications. It is preferable to dislodge the obstruction, rather than replace the tube (69). In order to minimize the risk of feeding tube obstruction 1) provide medications in the form of elixirs, rather than pills, if they are to be delivered via the feeding tube; 2) flush the tube with water or saline before and after medication administration; and 3) flush tube with water or saline after gastric residuals are checked (69). Once a tube is clogged, there have been several methods recommended to clear the obstruction. Irrigation from a syringe filled with warm water can be attempted (61). A mixture of pancreatic enzyme and sodium bicarbonate has been recommended to dissolve clots, using a smaller tube to deliver the mixture to the obstruction (53). When the obstruction is caused by a kinked or knotted tubing, the tube must either be repositioned or removed (61).

Pressure necrosis of the skin is caused by the feeding tube pressing against the mucosal surface. It may also result in mucosal ulceration, abscess formation, and perforation. The risk of pressure necrosis can be reduced by the use of small-bore soft feeding tubes or by replacing nasoenteric tubes with gastrostomy/jejunostomy tubes for long-term nutrition.

Leakage of the feeding tube contents can be a result of several problems. In the case of a dysfunctional tube, the tube should be replaced. If leakage is secondary to an infection, antibiotic therapy, debridement, and/or feeding tube removal may be indicated. Stomal enlargement is also a reason for tube leakage and can be treated by decreasing the diameter of the stoma and then replacing the tube.

Gastrointestinal (61)

Regurgitation occurs when the feeding formula is not absorbed and consequently accumulates and backs up in the gastrointestinal tract. The feedings should be held or decreased while establishing the cause of the problem. Aspiration may result as a complication of regurgitation. The risk of aspiration is reduced by elevating the head of the bed, placement of blocks under the head of the bed, regularly checking gastric residuals, using small-bore feeding tubes, providing feedings via continuous delivery, and placing the feeding tube beyond the pyloric sphincter. Although difficult, residuals could be checked with a large syringe (60 cc or greater). The smaller the syringe, the greater the hydrolic advantage and the likelihood that the tube will collapse. In some instances, it may be desirable to feed transpylorically (eg, into the small bowel) while decompressing the stomach with a temporary or permanent gastric tube.

Diarrhea is one of the most common gastrointestinal complications associated with enteral nutrition. However, it is usually not a result of the tube feeding itself (69). If the gastrointestinal tract is part of the field during radiation therapy, radiation enteritis may be a result. Also, surgery to various parts of the gastrointestinal tract may lead to diarrhea (e.g. dumping syndrome after gastric resection, fat maldigestion, and malabsorption after small bowel resection).

Some antibiotics may effect opportunistic proliferation of pathogenic organisms normally suppressed by competitive organisms in the GI tract. The result is diarrhea caused by the decreased absorption and increased secretion of fluid and electrolytes. Clostridium difficile, the organism most often associated with antibiotic-related diarrhea, accounts for 10 percent to 25 percent of all cases. Clostridium perfingens, Salmonella, Shigella, Campylobacter, Yersinia enterocolitica, and Escheria coli organisms have also been implicated (61).

Diarrhea can also be caused by overfeeding, hypoalbuminemia, osmotically active medications, and microbial contamination of the feeding product. Especially in a compromised patient, the administration of a contaminated formula can result in diarrhea, pneumonia, and septicemia.

Constipation may also occur during enteral nutrition. Certain types of chemotherapeutic agents may result in constipation as a side effect (2). A non-pharmacotherapeutic remedy for this problem can be the use of fiber-containing formulas. Also, the adequate provision of water (see Chapter 4, *Calorie, Protein, Fluid, and Micronutrient Requirements*) is important in preventing constipation in any patient, especially when using fiber-containing formulas.

Metabolic

The refeeding syndrome is a common metabolic complication of tube feeding delivery. It is caused by the rapid repletion of potassium, phosphorous, and magnesium. This occurs as these minerals move intracellularly with refeeding. It is more frequently seen in the severely malnourished or cachectic patient. The electrolyte abnormalities created by refeeding may result in generalized muscle weakness, tetany, cardiac dysfunction, seizures, arrhythmias, excess sodium and water retention, hemolytic anemia, phagocyte dysfunction, and death from cardiac or respiratory failure. The likelihood of refeeding syndrome can be minimized by taking two days to three days to reach nutritional goals in malnourished patients and providing a maintenance (or repletion, if needed) supply of potassium, phosphorous, and magnesium.

Dehydration, hypernatremia, and azotemia may occur during enteral feeding. These are most likely to occur in the unconscious or debilitated patient who cannot communicate or alleviate thirst. This is why it is important to not only provide calorie and protein requirements, but fluid needs as well (see Chapter 4, *Calorie, Protein, Fluid, and Micronutrient Requirements*, on nutritional goals).

Drug-nutrient interactions may occur during enteral nutrition. They are characterized by any change in the enteral formula or medication when the two are mixed (70). The review of medications for potential drug-nutrient interactions may help prevent this complication from occurring.

Transition to Oral Intake

If possible, the patient should be transitioned from enteral nutrition to oral intake. If the reason for enteral nutrition is dysphagia, this transition may be facilitated by a swallowing evaluation that is done by a speech/language pathologist. Calorie counts are often used to monitor oral intake. If a patient is consuming less than 1/2 of his or her nutrient requirements, tube feedings should be continued. Nocturnal feedings may be employed in order to stimulate daytime oral intake. Tube feedings can usually be discontinued if a patient is meeting 2/3 to 3/4 of his or her requirements by mouth. Deficits can be made up through the use of oral nutritional supplements.

Transition to Home

Discharge plans should be considered at the initiation of therapy (eg, whether short-term or long-term enteral support is indicated). Careful planning and instruction are necessary in order to ensure safe and effective therapy in the home setting. This is best accomplished through a multi-disciplinary approach. A reputable home care provider who communicates regularly with the team is essential. The time required to train patients will depend upon the therapy required and the patient's ability to learn. The patients must also be physically capable of performing the procedures. For the home enteral patients, actual training time will average between two to five hours over two to five days, once tolerance to the feeding is established. Patients should be provided with complete written instructions prior to discharge.

Palliative Care

For patients experiencing unsuccessful treatment, enteral nutrition may still be provided as a supportive measure providing nourishment, fluid, and electrolytes. The least aggressive and non-invasive means should be used in order to enhance patient care and comfort. It is the responsibility of the interdisciplinary team to inform the patient and family of the risks and benefits of enteral nutrition.

Summary

Enteral nutrition support, whether it be oral or via a feeding tube, remains the preferred method of nutrition delivery. Malnourished cancer patients may receive the benefits of preservation of gut integrity, decreased risk of infectious complications, and the relatively less expensive cost compared to parenteral nutrition. These benefits are in addition to the overall goal of nutrition support reversing or lessening the progression of malnutrition in the cancer patient.

References

1. Harrison LE, Fong Y. Enteral nutrition in the cancer patient. In: Rombeau JL, Rolandelli RH, eds. *Enteral and Tube Feeding.* Philadelphia, Pa: W.B. Saunders; 1997:300-323.
2. Bloch AS. Cancer. In: Matarese LE, Gottschlich MM, eds. *Contemporary Nutrition Support Practice.* Philadelphia, Pa: W.B. Saunders Company; 1998:475-495.
3. Steiger E, Oram-Smith J, Miller E, Kuo L, Vars HM. Effects of nutrition on tumor growth and tolerance to chemotherapy. *J Surg Res.* 1975;18(4):455-461.
4. Alexander JW. Nutrition and translocation. *JPEN.* 1990;14(suppl):40S-44S.
5. Kudsk KA, Croce MA, Fabian TC, et al. Enteral versus parenteral feeding: Effects on septic morbidity after blunt and penetrating abdominal trauma. *Ann Surg.* 1992;215:503-513.
6. Moore FA, Moore EE, Jones TN, et al. TEN vs TPN following major abdominal trauma-reduced septic morbidity. *J Trauma.* 1989;29:916-923.
7. Bower RH, Talamini MA, Sax HC, et al. Prospective enteral vs. parenteral nutrition: A randomized control trial. *Arch Surg.* 1986;121: 040-1045.
8. Moore FA, Feliciano DV, Andrassy RJ, et al. Early enteral feeding, compared with parenteral, reduces postoperative septic complications. The results of a meta-analysis. *Ann Surg.* 1992;216:172-183.
9. Kudsk KA. Gut mucosal nutritional support-enteral nutrition as primary therapy after multiple system trauma. *Gut.* 1994;35:S52-S54.
10. Herndon DN, Barrow RE, Stein M, et al. Increased mortality with intravenous supplememtal feeding in severely burned patients. *J Burn Care Rehabil.* 1989;10:309-313.
11. Suchner V, Senftleben U, Eckart T, et al. Enteral versus parenteral nutrition: Effects on gastrointestinal function and metabolism. *Nutrition.* 1996;12:13-22.
12. Kudsk KA, Minard G, Wojtysiak SL, et al. Visceral protein response to enteral versus parenteral nutrition and sepsis in patients with trauma. *Surgery.* 1994;116:516-523.
13. Peterson VM, Moore EE, Jones TN, et al. Total enteral nutrition vs. total parenteral nutrition after major torso injury: Attenuation of hepatic protein reprioritization. *Surgery.* 1988;104:199-207.
14. Sedman PC, MacFie J, Palmer MD, Mitchell CJ, Sagar PM. Preoperative total parenteral nutrition is not associated with mucosal atrophy or bacterial translocation in humans. *Br J Surg.* 1995;82:1663-1666.
15. Moore EE, Jones TN. Benefits of immediate jejunostomy feeding after major abdominal trauma: A prospective randomized trial. *J Trauma.* 1986;26:874-881.
16. Kudsk KA, Carpenter G, Peterson S, Sheldon GF. Effect of enteral and parenteral feeding in malnourished rats with E. coli-hemoglobin adjuvant peritonitis. *J Surg Res.* 1981;31:105-110.
17. Saito H, Trocki O, Alexander JW, et al. The effect of route of nutrient administration on the nutritional state, catabolic hormone secretion, and gut mucosal integrity after burn injury. *JPEN.* 1987;11:1-7.
18. Alverdy JC, Aoys E, Moss GS. Total parenteral nutrition promotes bacterial translocation from the gut. *Surgery.* 1988;104:185-190.

19. Delaney HM, John J, Tek EL, et al. Contrasting effects of identical nutrients given parenterally or enterally after 70% hepatectomy. *J Surg* .1994;167:135-144.
20. Pappo I, Polacheck I, Zmora O, et al. Altered gut barrier function to Candida during paraenteral nutrition. *Nutrition.* 1994;10:151-154.
21. Mainous M, Xu D, Lu Q, et al. Ora-TPN-induced bacterial translocation and impaired immune defenses are reversed by refeeding. *Surgery.* 1991;110:277-284.
22. Waters B, Kudsk KA, Jarvi EJ, et al. Effect of route of nutrition on recovery of hepatic organic anion clearance after fasting. *Surgery.* 1994;115:370-374.
23. Langkamp-Henken B, Glezer JA, Kudsk KA. Immunologic structure and function of the gastrointestinal tract. *Nutr Clin Pract.* 1992;7:100-108.
24. Newsholme EA, Crabtree B, Ardawi MS. Glutamine metabolism in lymphocytes: Its biochemical, physiological and clinical importance. *Q J Exp Physiol.* 1985;70:473-489.
25. Kovacevic Z, Morris HP. The role of glutamine in the oxidative metabolism of malignant cells. *Cancer Res.* 1972;32:326-333.
26. Lacey JM, Wilmore DW. Is glutamine a conditionally essential amino acid? *Nutr Rev.* 1990;48:297-309.
27. Ziegler TR, Smith RJ, Byrne TA, et al. Potential role of glutamine supplementation in nutrition support. *Clin Nutr.* 1993;12(suppl 1):S82-S90.
28. Buchman AL, Moukarzel AA, Ament ME, et al. Parenteral nutriton leads to a decrease in intestinal mucosal thickness and an increase in intestinal permeability in man. *Gastroenterology.* 1993;104: A612. Abstract.
29. Young LS, Stoll S. Protein in Nutrition Support. In: Matarese LE, Gottschlich MM, eds. *Contemporary Nutrition Support.* Philadelphia Pa: W.B. Saunders; 1998:97-109.
30. Ziegler TR, Smith RJ, Byrne TA, et al. Potential role of glutamine supplementation in nutrition support. *Clin Nutr.* 1993;12(suppl 1):S82-S90.
31. Stehle P, Mertes N, Puchstein CH, et al. Effect of parenteral glutamine peptide supplements on muscle glutamine loss and nutrogen balance after major surgery. *Lancet.* 1989;1:231-233.
32. Furst P, Albers S, Stehle P. Glutamine-containing dippeptides in parenteral nutrition. *JPEN.* 1990;14(suppl 4):118S-124S.
33. Vinnars E, Hammarqvist F, von der Decken A, et al. Role of glutamine and its analogs in posttraumatic muscle protein and amino acid metabolism. *JPEN.* 1990;14:125S-129S.
34. Hammarqvist F, Wernerman J, Ali R, et al. Addition of glutamine to total parenteral nutrition after elective abdominal surgery spares free glutamine in muscle, counteracts the fall in muscle protein synthesis, and improves nitrogen balance. *Ann Surg.* 1989;209:455-461.
35. Wernerman J, Hammarqvist F, Ali MR. Glutamine and ornithine-alpha-ketoglutarate but not branched chain amino acids reduce the loss of muscle glutamine after surgical trauma. *Metabolism.* 1989;38:63-66.
36. Van der Hulst RRW, Van Kreel BK, et al. Glutamine and the preservation of gut integrity. *Lancet.* 1993;341:1363-1365.
37. Tremel H, Kienle B, Weilemann LS, et al. Glutamine dipeptide supplemented TPN maintains intestinal function in the critically ill. *Gastroenterology.* 1994;107:1595-1601.
38. Ziegler TR, Young LS, Benfell K, et al. Clinical and metabolic efficiency of glutamine-supplemented parenteral nutrition after bone marrow transplantation. A randomized, double-blind, controlled study. *Ann Intern Med.* 1992;116:821-828.
39. Schloeb PR, Amare M. Total parenteral nutrition with glutamine in bone marrow transplantation and other clinical applications (a randomized, double-blind study). *JPEN.* 1993;17:407-413.
40. MacBurney M, Young LS, Ziegler TR, et al. A cost-evaluation of glutamine-supplemented parenteral nutrition in adult bone marrow transplantation. *J Am Diet Assoc.* 1994;94:1263-1266.
41. Kripke SA, Fox AD, Berman JM, Settle RG, Rombeau JL. Stimulation of intestinal mucosal growth with intracolonic infusion of short-chain fatty acids. *JPEN.* 1989;13:109-116.
42. Scheppach W, Bartram P, Richter A, Liepold G, Dussel H, Kasper MD. The effect of short-chain fatty acids on cecal crypt proliferation in man *JPEN.* 1990;14(suppl):12S. Abstract.
43. Slavin JL, Nelson NL, McNamara EA, Cashmere K. Bowel function of healthy men consuming liquid diets with and without dietary fiber. *JPEN.* 1985;9(3):317-321.
44. Frankenfield DC, Beyer PL. Soy-polysaccharide fiber: Effect on diarrhea in tube-fed, head-injured patients. *Am J Clin Nutr.* 1989;50(3):533-538.

45. Tucker DM, Sandstead HH, Logan GM, et al. Dietary fiber and personality factors as determinants of stool output. *Gastroenterology.* 1981;81(5):879-883.

46. Evans MA, Shronts EP. Intestinal fuels: Glutamine, short chain fatty acids, and dietary fiber. *J Am Diet Assoc.* 1992;92(10):1239-1246.

47. Heymsfield SB, Roongspisuthipong C, Evert M, et al. Fiber supplementation of enteral formulas: Effect on the bioavailability of major nutrients and gastrointestinal tolerance. *JPEN.* 1988;12(3):265-273.

48. Spiegel JE, Rose R, Karabell P, Frankos VH, Schmitt DF. Safety and benefits of fructooligosaccharides as food ingredients. *Food Technol.* 1994;48(1):85-89.

49. DeChicco RS, Matarese LE. Determining the nutrition support regimen. In: Matarese LE, Gottschlich MM, eds. *Contemporary Nutrition Support Practice.* Philadelphia, Pa: W.B. Saunders; 1998:185-191.

50. Gottschlich MM. Early and perioperative nutrition support. In: Matarese LE, Gottschlich MM, eds. *Contemporary Nutrition Support Practice.* Philadelphia, Pa: W.B. Saunders; 1998:279-292.

51. Kudsk KA. Clinical applications of enteral nutrition. *Nutr Clin Pract.* 1994;9:165-171.

52. Klein S, Koretz RL. Nutrition support in patients with cancer: what do the data really show? *Nutr Clin Pract.* 1994;9:91-100.

53. Tchekmedyian NS. Costs and benefits of nutrition support in cancer. *Oncology.* 1995;9(11 suppl):79-84.

54. Tchmedyian NS. Pharmacoeconomics of nutritional support in cancer. *Seminars in Oncology* 1998; 25 (2 Suppl 6): 62-69.

55. Hummell AC, Bloch AS, MacInnis P, Winkler MF. *Clinical Indicator Wokbook for Nutrition Care Systems.* Chicago, Ill: American Dietetic Association; 1994.

56. Burt ME, Brennan MF. Nutritional support of the patient with esophageal cancer. *Semin Oncol.* 1984;11(2):127.

57. Kokal WA. The impact of antitumor therapy on nutrition. *Cancer.* 1985; 55:273.

58. McArdle AH, Wittnich C, Freeman CR. Elemental diet as prophylaxis against radiation injury: histologic and ultrastructural studies. *Arch Surg.* 1985;120:1026.

59. Trujillo EB, Enteral nutrition: a comprehensive overview. In Matarese LE, Gottschlich MM, eds. *Contemporary Nutrition Support Practice.* Philadelphia, Pa: W.B. Saunders; 1998:192-201.

60. Gottschlich MM, Shronts EP, Hutchins AM. Defined formula diets. In: Rombeau JL, Rolandelli RH, eds, *Enteral and Tube Feeding.* Philadelphia, Pa: W.B. Saunders; 1997:207-239.

61. Beyer PL. Complications of enteral nutrition. In: Matarese LE, Gottschlich MM, eds. *Contemporary Nutrition Support Practice.* Philadelphia, Pa: W.B. Saudners; 1998: 216-226.

62. Minard G. Enteral access. *Nutr Clin Pract.* 1994;9:172-182.

63. Lightdale CJ, Shike M, Bloch AS. *Gastrointestinal Endoscopy Clinics of North America.* Philadelphia, Pa: W.B. Saunders; 1998.

64. Clevenger FW, Rodriquez DJ. Decision-making for enteral feeding administration: the why behind where and how. *Nutr Clin Pract.* 1995;10:104-113.

65. Shike M, Latkany L. Direct percutaneous endoscopic jejunostomy. In: Lightdale C, Shike M, Bloch AS, eds. *Gastrointestinal Endoscopy Clinics of North America.* Philadelphia, Pa: W.B. Saunders; 1998:569-580.

66. Rombeau JL, Caldwell MD. *Enteral and Tube Feeding.* Philadelphia, Pa: W.B. Saunders; 1984.

67. Ideno KT. Enteral Nutrition. In: Gottschlich MM, Matarese LE, Shronts EP. *Nutrition Support Dietetics Core Curriculum.* Gaithersburg, Md: ASPEN; 1993:71-104.

68. Skipper A. *Dietitian's Handbook of Enteral and Parenteral Nutrition,* 2nd ed. Gaithersburg, Md: ASPEN; 1998.

69. Hamaoui E, Kodsi R. Complications of enteral feeding and their prevention. In: Rombeau JL, Rolandelli RH, eds. *Enteral and Tube Feeding.* Philadelphia, Pa: W.B. Saunders; 1997:554-574.

70. Rollins CJ. General Pharmacologic issues. In: Matarese LE, Gottschlich MM, eds. *Contemporary Nutrition Support Practice.* Philadelphia, Pa: W.B. Saunders; 1998:303-323.

12

Parenteral Nutrition in Medical/Surgical Oncology

Robert S. DeChicco, MS, RD, CNSD　　　**Ezra Steiger, MD, FACS, CNSP**

Malnutrition associated with cancer is characterized by weight loss, decreased serum proteins, impaired immunocompetence, and a poor prognosis (1-3). Parenteral nutrition (PN) is administered to oncology patients with the intent of improving nutritional status in order to increase the response rate to therapy and decrease morbidity and mortality. This is done despite the lack of clear evidence that PN improves outcomes in this population. Prior to administering PN to patients with cancer, the potential benefits must be balanced against the cost of the therapy and potential adverse consequences such as infectious complications and increased tumor growth.

Indications/Contraindications for PN

The decision to administer PN should be determined by the patient's disease status, gastrointestinal (GI) function, level of stress, and degree of malnutrition. Enteral nutrition support is preferable to PN since it provides nutrients in a less invasive, more cost efficient manner and helps preserve nutritional status and gut integrity with less risk of infectious complications (4,5). However, PN is a viable therapy in patients who are unable to tolerate nutrition via the gut. Indications for PN include a nonfunctional GI tract, the need for bowel rest, or severe malnutrition or catabolism when the patient is unable to eat for at least five days (Box 12.1). Contraindications for PN include a functional GI tract, inability to obtain intravenous (IV) access, a poor prognosis not warranting aggressive nutrition support, and when therapy is needed for less than five days in patients without severe stress or malnutrition.

Box 12.1　Indications for Parenteral Nutrition

Nonfunctional GI tract
- Severe diarrhea/malabsorption
- Short bowel syndrome
- Intractable nausea/vomiting
- Bowel obstruction or ileus

Need for bowel rest
- Severe pancreatitis
- Enterocutaneous fistula
- Exacerbation of Crohn's disease or ulcerative colitis

Effect of PN on Nutritional Status and Outcomes

Parenteral nutrition is effective in improving nutritional indices in patients with cancer, but its effect on clinical outcome is not clear. Parenteral nutrition has been associated with increases in weight, body fat, and visceral proteins in patients receiving chemotherapy (6-9) or radiation therapy (10-12). Unfortunately, most studies have been unable to demonstrate a consistent increase in lean body mass (7,13-16). Several investigations have demonstrated a significant reduction in postoperative complications such as wound infections in patients receiving perioperative PN for at least seven days (17-20). In some studies, the only patients who benefited from PN were in the group considered to be the most malnourished (17,20). In other cases, PN either had no effect (21,22) or has been associated with an increased incidence of complications (23), decreased survival (14,24), and decreased duration of remission (6) in patients receiving chemotherapy, radiation therapy, or surgery. The one population in which PN appears to positively affect long-term survival is patients undergoing bone marrow transplants (25).

Parenteral nutrition has also been administered in an attempt to decrease antineoplastic therapy-related toxicities such as leukopenia, thereby allowing more aggressive treatment and improved response rates, but the data is not conclusive (15,24,26). Parenteral nutrition can stimulate tumor growth in animals (27,28) but this has not been supported by in vivo studies in humans (14,17).

Practical Aspects of Administering PN

The goal of PN is to provide the patient's nutritional requirements in a safe and efficacious manner. The clinician must understand the components of the PN solution and techniques of administration to maximize the benefits while minimizing the potential adverse consequences of the therapy.

Macronutrients

The macronutrients used in PN solutions are carbohydrate in the form of dextrose, fat in the form of lipid emulsions, and protein in the form of amino acids (Table 12.1). The amounts of macronutrients are based on the clinical status and nutritional requirements of the patient. Dextrose is generally the best tolerated and least expensive source of IV calories. The minimum carbohydrate requirement for an adult is 100 grams/day to 150 grams/day. The maximum dextrose infusion rate should not exceed 5 mg/kg/minute (29). Lipids are not only a source of calories, but also provide essential fatty acids (EFAs). The optimal intake of IV fat is not known, but requirements for EFAs can be met by providing at least 3% of total calories as lipids (30). This can be accomplished by admixing fat with the PN solution or by infusing 500 mL of 20% fat emulsion once per week. Amino acid solutions are available as a standard mixture of essential and nonessential amino acids or in disease-specific formulas for patients in acute renal failure or with hepatic encephalopathy.

Table 12.1   Macronutrients in PN Solutions

	Kcal/gram	Availability
Dextrose	3.4	5%–70%
Lipids	9.0	10%–30%
Amino acids	4.0	3%–15%

Electrolytes

Electrolytes are added daily to the PN solution to maintain electrolyte homeostasis. Electrolyte requirements vary among individuals based on clinical status, renal function, and pharmacotherapy (Table 12.2). In addition to maintenance requirements, it is necessary to replace electrolytes lost via the GI tract due to fistulas, high-output ostomies, or persistent vomiting or diarrhea. Reviewing the patient's maintenance IV fluids prior to starting PN may help estimate electrolyte requirements. However, it is important to understand that, in general, PN will increase electrolyte requirements, particularly potassium, magnesium, and phosphorus in order to support anabolism. See Chapter 4, *Calorie, Protein, Fluid, and Micronutrient Requirements*, for a discussion of fluid requirements.

Table 12.2   Daily Intravenous Electrolyte Requirements for Adults with Normal Renal Function (35)

Electrolytes	Usual Adult IV Dose
Sodium	100–150 mEq
Potassium	60–120 mEq
Chloride	100–150 mEq
Magnesium	8–24 mEq
Phosphorus	15–30 mmol

Source: *The Cleveland Clinic Foundation Nutrition Support Handbook,* Cleveland, Ohio. Used with permission.

Vitamins/Trace Elements

Vitamins and trace elements are essential for normal metabolism and cellular function and should be added to PN solutions daily. Intravenous requirements for vitamins and trace elements were established by the Nutrition Advisory Group of the American Medical Association Department of Foods and Nutrition (31,32) (Table 12.3). Since the original recommendations, there has also been evidence to support the addition of selenium to PN solutions (33). It is common practice to add up to 120 mcg selenium/d. It is important to be aware of the content of multivitamin and trace element solutions. Many multivitamin solutions do not contain vitamin K due to potential interference with anticoagulation therapy. Multi-trace element solutions can contain anywhere from four to six components. Vitamins and trace elements can be added as single entities if needed.

Table 12.3   Parenteral Vitamin and Trace Element Requirements for Adults (31,32)

Vitamins	Requirements
A (IU)	3300
D (IU)	200
E (IU)	10
Ascorbic acid (mg)	100
Folic acid (mcg)	400
Niacin (mg)	40
Riboflavin (mg)	3.6
Thiamin (mg)	3.0
B6 (mg)	4.0
B12 (mcg)	5.0
Pantothenic acid (mg)	15
Biotin (mcg)	60
Trace elements	
Chromium (mcg)	10–15
Copper (mg)	0.5–1.5
Manganese (mcg)	150–800
Zinc (mg) *	2.5–4.0

*Add 2.0 mg for catabolism, 12.2 mg/L small bowel fluid loss, 17.1 mg/kg stool loss

Medications

The use of PN as a vehicle for administering medications is generally not recommended due to potential incompatibility between the drug and the component of the solution, the inability to titrate the drug or discontinue the dose without discontinuing the solution, and the necessity to infuse medications continuously rather than intermittently. Nonetheless, certain medications are routinely added to PN solutions including heparin, insulin, and H2 blockers. Other medications that have been added to PN solutions include antibiotics, aminophylline, metoclopramide, octreotide, and steroids. Potential advantages of using PN solutions to deliver medications include cost savings due to decreased use of materials and labor, fluid savings due to a decrease in IVs, and a lower risk of contamination due to less manipulation of the IV lines. A pharmacist should be consulted before adding any medication to a PN solution.

Formula Selection—Peripheral versus Central

The type of PN formula is determined by the clinical and nutritional status of the patient along with the type of IV access (Box 12.2). Patients with cancer usually have central IV access to accommodate multiple IV therapies. When central IV access is not available, PN can be infused via a peripheral catheter. Peripheral PN requires a formula that is modest in osmolarity and periodic changing of IV sites to prevent thrombophlebitis. Peripheral formulas are generally lipid-based and moderate in protein since dextrose and amino acids are more osmotically active than fat. Peripheral PN solutions with a final dextrose concentration of 10% or less and an osmolarity below 900 mOsm/kg are generally well-tolerated by peripheral veins. Since peripheral PN may be limited in dextrose and protein, it is appropriate for patients who are mildly stressed or malnourished.

Central PN solutions are not limited by osmolarity since they are infused through a larger vein. Therefore, central solutions can be concentrated and are appropriate in patients who are severely stressed and hypermetabolic or require a fluid restriction. Central solutions can be either lipid- or dextrose-based. Dextrose-based solutions are preferred in patients who can tolerate the carbohydrate load, thereby avoiding compatibility and immunosuppression concerns associated with IV fats. Lipid-based solutions are appropriate when minimizing carbohydrate intake is desirable due to hyperglycemia or hypercapnia.

Box 12.2   Indications for Peripheral and Central PN

Peripheral
  Short term (ie, <5–7 days)
  Mild to moderate malnutrition
  Normal to mildly increased metabolic rate
  No fluid restriction

Central
  Long term (ie, >7 days)
  Moderate to severe malnutrition
  Moderately to severely stressed
  Fluid restriction
  Poor peripheral access
  Allergy to IV lipids

Administration Techniques

Parenteral nutrition is usually administered continuously in the hospital because it requires less effort and manipulation of the IV lines and is easier to manage fluid and electrolytes. When initiating PN, the patient should receive one half of the desired calories for the first 24 hours to allow the patient time to adjust to the carbohydrate load. If the patient tolerates the PN at half calories, the calories (and carbohydrate) can be advanced. For patients on long-term therapy or going home or to a nursing facility, PN is usually cycled over 8 hours to 16 hours to allow time away from the infusion pump and IV pole. Cycling may also help prevent cholestasis and elevated liver function tests (34). The usual method used to cycle PN is to subtract four hours each day from the administration time until the desired cycle length is achieved or the patient cannot tolerate the fluid or carbohydrate load.

Tapering (ie, gradually increasing or decreasing the infusion rate at the beginning or end of the cycle) is used to prevent severe changes in blood glucose due to the abrupt infusion or discontinuation of carbohydrate. Tapering helps the patient avoid hyperglycemia at the beginning of the cycle and rebound hypoglycemia at the end of the cycle.

Monitoring

Monitoring patients during PN infusion will help prevent PN-associated complications and assess nutritional status and the efficacy of therapy. Serum levels of electrolytes, blood urea nitrogen, and creatinine should be monitored daily for the first several days after the initiation of PN and then less frequently once the patient is stable (Table 12.4). Blood sugars should be checked every six hours until the patient is stable on PN providing full calories. The patient's weight, fluid intake and output, and vital signs should be reviewed daily. Nutritional parameters such as visceral proteins, nitrogen balance, and anthropometrics can be determined weekly since there is little change from day to day. Trace elements including copper, selenium, manganese, chromium, and zinc should be checked every six months in patients on home PN (35).

Table 12.4   Monitoring Guidelines for PN (35)

Parameter	Frequency
Serum sodium, potassium, chloride, CO2, calcium, phosphorus, magnesium, creatinine, blood urea nitrogen	Daily for at least first three days, then less often in stable patients
Serum glucose	Accuchecks every six hours initially, then less often in stable patients
Liver function tests	Weekly
Visceral proteins (albumin, transferrin, or prealbumin)	Weekly
Fluid intake/output	Daily during duration of therapy
Vital signs	Daily during duration of therapy
Weight	Daily initially, then less often in stable patients

Complications

Complications associated with PN can be categorized as mechanical (e.g. subclavian vein thrombosis, pneumothorax, catheter tip misplacement), infectious (e.g. catheter-related sepsis), and metabolic (e.g. hyperglycemia, hypokalemia, elevated liver function tests). Careful patient monitoring, catheter care, and formula preparation and administration will help prevent complications. Hyperglycemia, the most common metabolic complication of PN, can be treated by adding insulin and/or decreasing the amount of carbohydrate infused. Insulin should be added directly to the PN rather than administered subcutaneously since it is easier to control blood sugars when both the carbohydrate and insulin are administered continuously. Carbohydrate intake can be decreased by limiting total calories or by replacing dextrose with fat calories. Hypoglycemia is usually caused by excess insulin or by abrupt discontinuation of the PN solution. If PN needs to be stopped immediately, it should be replaced by D_{10} for one hour. If time allows, PN should be decreased to half rate for one hour before discontinuing.

Home Parenteral Nutrition

Cancer is the most common diagnosis in patients on home PN the United States (36). Indications for home PN are the same as those used in an acute care setting. However, due to the length and complexity of home PN, the patient must also meet additional criteria to be considered a candidate. The patient must be medically and emotionally stable and have a relatively long life expectancy (ie, > six months). The patient must be able to perform the tasks associated with home PN or have a primary caregiver who is available during the time the solution is infusing. The patient must have a long-term IV access device in place and be on a stable PN formula prior to discharge. There must be a program in place to monitor the patient and deal with complications after discharge. The patient's need for home PN should be reviewed periodically.

Transition to Enteral Feedings

One of the primary goals for patients on PN, whenever possible, is to wean from IV nutrition to nutrition via the GI tract. Enteral nutrition should be started as soon as the patient has adequate GI function. However, PN should not be discontinued until the patient has demonstrated the ability to digest, absorb, and utilize enteral nutrients in adequate amounts either orally, via a feeding tube, or in combination. When transitioning patients from PN to tube feedings (TFs), the PN can be decreased by one-half once TFs are at 33% to 50% of the goal rate. The PN can then be discontinued once TFs are advanced to greater than 75% of the goal rate (37). When transitioning from PN to oral feedings, PN can be decreased by one half once the patient is tolerating a diet advanced beyond clear liquids. PN can be discontinued once the patient is tolerating solid foods and taking adequate fluids to prevent dehydration.

Summary

The use of PN in patients with cancer is controversial. In the past, PN was routinely administered to malnourished patients with cancer who could not tolerate enteral feedings, but there is a lack of evidence to support this practice. Parenteral nutrition is effective in treating malnutrition associated with cancer (6–12), but does not improve response to anti-tumor therapy or decrease toxicities due to chemotherapy or radiation therapy (15,24,26). The inherent risks associated with PN such as increased risk of infection should also be weighed against the potential benefits. Therefore, PN should not be routinely administered to patients undergoing chemotherapy or radiation therapy who are unable to eat, but are expected to resume enteral nutrition within one week.

It was also fairly routine in the past to administer PN to cancer patients undergoing major surgical procedures. However, there is little evidence to suggest that perioperative PN improves surgical morbidity or mortality in patients who are not severely malnourished (20–22). In fact, surgical patients who receive PN, in some studies, had poorer outcomes than patients who received standard oral nutrition (23). Therefore, PN should not be administered to well-nourished or mildly malnourished patients undergoing surgery who are expected to resume enteral feedings within one week.

Prognosis must be considered when determining who should receive PN. Generally, PN is not indicated in patients with advanced cancer who are not responsive to anti-tumor therapy or in whom no therapy is planned. Parenteral nutrition exposes these patients to the risks of the therapy without increasing their quality of life or life expectancy.

Parenteral nutrition is appropriate in several subgroups of cancer patients. Parenteral nutrition appears to benefit patients with cancer undergoing chemotherapy or radiation therapy who are unable to tolerate enteral feedings for one week or longer. In severely malnourished patients undergoing surgery, preoperative PN can decrease postoperative morbidity and mortality when administered for at least seven days (17,20). Parenteral nutrition may also increase survival in patients undergoing bone marrow transplants (25). These guidelines are consistent with ones established by the American Society for Parenteral and Enteral Nutrition (ASPEN) for patients with cancer (38).

There is little evidence to support the widespread use of home PN in patients with cancer. Home PN is seldom indicated in patients with advanced cancer who are not being aggressively treated for their disease. Generally, these patients have progressive disease with poor response to anti-tumor therapies and a short life expectancy, with or without PN.

Home PN may be beneficial in oncology patients with gut dysfunction who are being aggressively treated and have demonstrated a positive response to anti-tumor therapy. Home PN may also benefit patients with slow-growing tumors who have a relatively long life expectancy.

References

1. Eastern Cooperative Oncology Group. Prognostic effect of weight loss prior to chemotherapy in cancer patients. *Am J Med.* 1980;69:491-497.

2. Nixon DW, Heymsfield SB, Cohen AE, Kutner MH, Ansley J, Lawson DH, Rudman D. Protein-calorie undernutrition in hospitaized cancer patients. *Am J Med.* 1980;68:683-690.

3. Smale BF, Mullen JL, Buzby GP, Rosato EF. The efficacy of nutritional assessment and support in cancer surgery. *Cancer.* 1981;47:2375-2381.

4. Kudsk KA, Croce MA, Fabian TC, Minard G, Tolley E, Poret A, Kuhl MR, Brown RO. Enteral versus parenteral feeding. Effects on septic morbidity after blunt and penetrating abdominal trauma. *Ann Surg.* 1992;215:503-511.

5. Moore FA, Moore EE, Jones TN, McCroskey BL, Peterson VM. TEN versus TPN following major abdominal trauma - reduced septic morbidity. *J Trauma.* 1989;29:916-922.

6. Shamberger RC, Brennan MF, Goodgame JT, Lowry SF, Maher MM, Wesley RA, Pizzo PA. A prospective, randomized study of adjuvant parenteral nutrition in the treatment of sarcomas: Results of metabolic and survival studies. *Surgery.* 1984;96:1-13.

7. Shike M, Russell D, Detsky AS, Harrison JE, McNeill KG, Shepherd FA, Feld R, Evans WK, Jeejeebhoy KN. Changes in body composition in patients with small-cell lung cancer. *Ann Intern Med.* 1984;101:303-309.

8. Smith RC, Hartemink R. Improvement of nutritional measures during preoperative parenteral nutrition in patients selected by the prognostic nutritional index: A randomized controlled trial. *JPEN.* 1988;12:587-591.

9. DeCicco M, Panarello G, Fantin D, Veronesi A, Pinto A, Zagonel V, Monfardini S, Testa V. Parenteral nutrition in cancer patients receiving chemotherapy: Effects on toxicity and nutritional status. *JPEN.* 1993;17:513-518.

10. Kinsella TJ, Malcolm AW, Bothe A, Valerio D, Blackburn GL. Prospective study of nutritional support during pelvic irradiation. *Int J Radiat Oncol Biol Phys.* 1981;7:543-548.

11. Burt ME, Gorschboth CM, Brennan MF. A controlled, prospective, randomized trial evaluating the metabolic effects of enteral and parenteral nutrition in the cancer patient. *Cancer.* 1982;49:1092-1105.

12. Burt ME, Stein TP, Brennan MF. A controlled randomized trial evaluating the effects of enteral and parenteral nutrition on protein metabolism in cancer-bearing man. *J Surg Res.* 1983;34:303-314.

13. Nixon DW, Lawson DH, Kutner M, Ansley J, Schwarz M, Heymsfield S, Chawla R, Cartwright TH, Rudman D. Hyperalimentation of the cancer patient with protein-calorie undernutrition. *Cancer Res.* 1981;41:2038-2045.

14. Nixon DW, Moffitt S, Lawson DH, Ansley J, Lynn MJ, Kutner MH, Heymsfield SB, Wesley M, Chawla R, Rudman D. Total parenteral nutrition as an adjunct to chemotherapy of metastatic colorectal cancer. *Cancer Treat Rep.* 1981;65:121-128.

15. Popp MB, Morrison SD, Brennan MF. Total parenteral nutrition in a methylcholanthrene-induced rat sarcoma model. *Cancer Treat Rep.* 1981;65:137-143.

16. Drott C, Unsgaard B, Schersten T, Lundholm K. Total parenteral nutrition as an adjuvant to patients undergoing chemotherapy for testicular carcinoma: Protection of body composition - a randomized, prospective trial. *Surgery.* 1988;103:499-506.

17. Mullen JL, Buzby GP, Matthews DC, Smale BF, Rosato EF. Reduction of operative morbidity and mortality by combined preoperative and postoperative nutritional support. *Ann Surg.* 1980;192:604-613.

18. Muller JM, Keller HW, Brenner U, Walter M, Holzmuller W. Indications and effects of preoperative parenteral nutrition. *W J Surg.* 1986;10:53-63.

19. Fan S, Lo C, Lai E, Chu K, Liu C, Wung J. Perioperative nutritional support in patients undergoing hepatectomy for hepatocellular carcinoma. *N Engl J Med.* 1994;331:1547-1552.

20. The Veterans Affairs Total Parenteral Nutrition Cooperative Study Group. Perioperative total parenteral nutrition in surgical patients. *N Engl J Med.* 1991;325:525-532.

21. Holter AR, Fischer JE. The effects of perioperative hyperalimentation on complications in patients with carcinoma and weight loss. *J Surg Res.* 1977;23:31-34.

22. Thompson BR, Julian TB, Stremple JF. Perioperative total parenteral nutrition in patients with gastrointestinal cancer. *J Surg Res.* 1981;30:497-500.

23. Brennan MF, Pisters P, Rosner M, Quesada O, Shike M. A prospective randomized trial of total parenteral nutrition after major pancreatic resection for malignancy. *Ann Surg.* 1994;220:436-444.

24. Jordan WM, Valdivieso M, Frankmann C, Gillespie M, Issell BF, Bodey GB, Freireich EJ. Treatment of advanced adenocarcinoma of the lung with Ftorafur, Doxorubicin, Cyclophosphamide, Cisplatin (FACP) and intensive IV hyperalimentation. *Cancer Treat Rep.* 1981;65:197-205.

25. Weisdorf SA, Lysne J, Wind D, Haake RJ, Sharp HL, Goldman A, Schissel K, McGlave PB, Ramsay NK, Kersey JH. Positive effect of prophylactic total parenteral nutrition on long-term outcome of bone marrow transplantation. *Transplantation.* 1987;43:833-838.

26. Weiner RS, Kromer BS, Clamon GH, Feld R, Evans W, Moran EM, Blum R, Weisenthal LM, Pee D, Hoffman FA, DeWys WD. Effects of intravenous hyperalimentation during treatment in patients with small cell lung cancer. *J Clin Oncol.* 1985;3:949-957.

27. Steiger E, Oram-Smith J, Miller E, Kuo L, Vars HM. Effects of nutrition on tumor growth and tolerance to chemotherapy. *J Surg Res.* 1975;18:455-461.

28. Daly JM, Copeland EM, Dudrick SJ. Effect of intravenous nutrition on tumor growth and host immunocompetence in malnourished animals. *Surgery.* 1978;84:655-658.

29. Wolfe RR, O'Donnell TF, Stone MD, Richmand DA, Burke JF. Investigation of factors determining the optimal glucose infusion rate in total parenteral nutrition. *Metab Clin Exp.* 1980;29:892-900.

30. Barr LH, Dunn GD, Brennan MF. Essential fatty acid deficiency during total parenteral nutrition. *Ann Surg.* 1981;193:304-311.

31. Multivitamin preparations for parenteral use: A statement by the Nutrition Advisory Group. *JPEN.* 1979;3:258-262.

32. Guidelines for essential trace element preparations for parenteral use: A statement by the Nutrition Advisory Group. *JPEN.* 1979;3:263-267.

33. Baptista RJ, Bistrian BR, Blackburn GL, Miller DG, Champagne CD, Buchanan L. Utilizing selenious acid to reverse selenium deficiency in total parenteral nutrition patients. *AJCN.* 1984;8:695-699.

34. Maini B, Blackburn GL, Bistrian BR, Flatt JP, Page JG, Bothe A, Benotti P, Reinhoff HY. Cyclic hyperalimentation: An optimal technique for preservation of visceral protein. *J Surg Res.* 1976:20:515-525.

35. Matarese LE (ed). The Cleveland Clinic Foundation Nutrition Support Handbook. Cleveland, Ohio: 1997; 52.

36. Howard L, Ament M, Fleming CR, Shike M, Steiger E. Current use and clinical outcome of home parenteral and enteral nutrition therapies in the United States. *Gastroenterol.* 1995;109:355-365.

37. Zibrida JM, Carlson SJ. Transitional feeding. In: Gottschlich MM, Matarese LE, Shronts EP, eds. *Nutrition Support Dietetics Core Curriculum.* Silver Spring, Md: ASPEN, 1993:459-466.

38. ASPEN Board of Directors. Guidelines for the use of parenteral and enteral nutrition in adult and pediatric patients. *JPEN.* 1993;17:12SA-13SA.

13

Pharmacological Management of Anorexia and Cachexia

Suellen Murphy, RN   Jamie H. Von Roenn, MD

Anorexia and cachexia are frequent clinical problems associated with cancer and human immunodeficiency (HIV) infection and ultimately affect the majority of patients with advanced disease. Cachexia refers to a multifactorial syndrome that is characterized by loss of appetite, generalized wasting, muscle atrophy, and a variety of metabolic abnormalities. Diagnosing and correcting the problems that may contribute to involuntary weight loss are the first steps in the management of anorexia (loss of appetite) and cachexia. Unfortunately, many patients experience weight loss without easily identifiable and/or reversible causes. A number of pharmacological agents have been examined to evaluate their impact on appetite, weight, and overall quality of life.

Dronabinol

Dronabinol, the primary orexigenic component of marijuana, has been shown to stimulate appetite in patients with acquired immunodeficiency syndrome (AIDS) and cancer-related anorexia (1–5). Results of studies conducted in cancer patients with weight loss and AIDS patients are highlighted below in Table 13.1.

Table 13.1   Dronabinol Trials

Patient Population	N	Treatment	↑ Appetite	Weight
Advanced cancer (2)	30	Dose ranging study 2.5 mg/d 2.5 mg BID 5 mg q day	In patients in 2 higher dose groups	↓ in rate of weight loss
Advanced cancer (3)	18	2.5 mg TID	13/18 patients	No weight change
AIDS (5)	89	Dronabinol 2.5 mg po BID vs placebo	19/50 patients	No weight change

N = number of patients

The only prospective randomized study of dronabinol for the treatment of cachexia enrolled patients with AIDS-related weight loss. Patients were randomized to either placebo or dronabinol, 2.5 mg orally, twice daily for 6 weeks. Patients treated with dronabinol had greater improvement in appetite and mood as compared to placebo-treated patients. There was no significant difference in weight between the treatment groups. After the 6 week study period, patients were offered treatment with dronabinol for up to 1 year. Available data from the 90 patients in the study extension demonstrates continued appetite stimulation for at least 6 months and body weight gain of 2 kg or more in 38% of patients (5).

Side Effects

Dizziness, euphoria, somnolence (drowsiness), and poor concentration have been reported as the most common side effects. Decreasing the dose may eliminate or lessen adverse effects.

Conclusion

Dronabinol, 2.5 mg po BID, can provide increased appetite as well as decreased nausea in patients with advanced cancer.

Megestrol Acetate

Megestrol acetate, a synthetic orally-active progestational agent used widely for the treatment of metastatic breast cancer, has been reported to stimulate appetite and weight gain. Treatment with conventional doses of megestrol acetate (160 mg/day) produces appetite stimulation and weight gain in about 30% of patients with advanced breast cancer (6). A phase I/II clinical trial of high-dose megestrol acetate (480 to 1600 mg/day) for the treatment of advanced breast cancer reported marked appetite stimulation and weight gain of more than 2 kgs in 81% of study participants (7). Subsequently, several placebo-controlled randomized studies have demonstrated the benefit of megestrol acetate for cancer-related cachexia as highlighted in Table 13.2.

Table 13.2   Cancer Cachexia Placebo-Controlled Trials of Megestrol Acetate (MA)

Author	N	MA Dose	Appetite	Weight
Loprinzi (8)	133	800 mg vs placebo	↑	Mean = 1.4 kg (MA group)
Bruera (9)	40	480 mg (cross over trial)	↑	
Tchekmedyian (10)	89	600 mg	↑	

N= number of patients

Across the studies, patients treated with megestrol acetate reported improved appetite, increased caloric intake and body weight and improved sense of well being. The beneficial effects of megestrol acetate on appetite and weight are dose dependent with greater benefit at higher doses.

Side Effects

Megestrol acetate can interfere with normal endocrine activities resulting in impotence in men, and infrequently, adrenal insufficiency or decreased glucose tolerance. The majority of randomized trials have failed to show a significant increase in either edema or deep vein thrombosis with megestrol acetate therapy.

Conclusion

For patients experiencing cancer-related cachexia, megestrol acetate 800 mg (20 cc of oral suspension) po q AM can provide significant weight gain and increased appetite. Megestrol acetate is available as 20 and 40 mg tablets or as an oral suspension (40mg/cc).

Corticosteroids

Numerous uncontrolled studies have advocated the use of corticosteroids for the treatment of cancer-related anorexia and cachexia. Multiple randomized placebo-controlled trials have demonstrated appetite enhancement with corticosteroid treatment (11–15). Table 13.3 highlights the results of these trials. In all of the studies, appetite improvement was short-lived (often < 8 weeks) and did not translate into weight gain.

Table 13.3 Corticosteroid Trials

Author	Steroid/Dose	Weight
Moertel (11)	Dexamethasone 0.75–1.5 mg po QID	No change
Wilcox (12)	Prednisolone 5 mg po TID	No change
Bruera (13)	Methylprednisolone 16 mg po BID	No change
Robustelli della Cuna (14)	Methylprednisolone 125 mg IV/d	No change
Popiela (15)	Methylprednisolone 125 mg IV/d	No change

In general, these trials enrolled patients with advanced cancer who were, as a result, treated with short courses (< 3 months) of treatment. In this advanced cancer population, improvement in appetite was associated with a self-reported improvement in quality of life.

Recently, the results of a comparative trial of dexamethasone, megestrol acetate, and fluoxymesterone (an anabolic agent) in patients with advanced cancer and weight loss have been reported. Four hundred and eighty patients were stratified on the basis of primary tumor site, weight loss in the preceding 2 months, planned concurrent therapy, performance status, and predicted survival (< 4 months, 4–6 months, > 6 months).

Patients were randomized to receive megestrol acetate 800 mg/day, dexamethasone 0.75 mg po QID or fluoxymesterone 10 mg po BID. Patient characteristics were well-balanced across the treatment groups. Median time on study was about 2 months. Over the relatively brief period of treatment, appetite stimulation and weight gain was not significantly different for patients treated with megestrol acetate or dexamethasone, but was significantly better than treatment with fluoxymesterone (16). All three drugs were reasonably well tolerated.

Side Effects

Prolonged use of corticosteroids may result in proximal muscle weakness, osteoporosis, delirium, fluid retention, adrenal suppression, glucose intolerance, and electrolyte disturbances.

Conclusion

For patients with very advanced cancer and limited survival (< 3 months) corticosteroids may provide palliation of anorexia. For bedridden patients, in particular, corticosteroids may be useful as exacerbation of muscle wasting is not of particular concern. Corticosteroids may be a particularly good therapy choice for patients who require co-analgesia with an anti-inflammatory agent (eg, the patient with painful bone metastases). Although clear dosing guidelines are not available from the published trials, dexamethasone, 4 mg every morning is a reasonable initial dose. An antacid or H_2 blocker (such as cimetidine) should be given concomitantly to avoid gastric irritation. Use of corticosteroids after 12 PM should be avoided because of the potential for insomnia.

Cyproheptadine

Cyproheptadine is an anti-serotonergic, antihistamine approved in the U.S. for the treatment of allergic disorders. In geriatric patients, adults with essential anorexia and adolescents with anorexia nervosa, cyproheptadine has been reported to improve appetite and stimulate weight gain. Two controlled trials, one in patients with advanced cancer and one in patients with AIDS-related weight loss have prospectively evaluated the nutritional impact of cyproheptadine (17,18) Results are shown in Table 13.4.

Table 13.4   Randomized Trials of Cyproheptadine

Author	Patient Population	Dose	Weight
Kardinal (17)	Adv. Cancer (n = 295)	8 mg po TID	No change
Summerbell (18)	AIDS (n = 14)	12 mg po/day	↑ 3.1 kg (mean)

Although the small study of cyproheptadine in patients with HIV-related weight loss reported an increase in weight (mean weight gain of 3.1 kg), the larger trial in advanced cancer patients was unable to demonstrate clear improvement in weight or appetite. As with other trials of treatment for anorexia and cachexia in advanced cancer patients, the time on therapy in the Kardinal study was brief; 75% of patients discontinued treatment before 3 months due to clinical deterioration.

Side Effects

Cyproheptadine is well-tolerated overall. Because of its atropine-like action, it should be used with caution in patients with asthma, increased intraocular pressure, hyperthyroidism, cardiac disease, and hypertension. Cyproheptadine may cause drowsiness, dry mouth, or difficulty with urination.

Conclusions

Because of its limited efficacy, cyproheptadine cannot be recommended for the treatment of cancer-related anorexia.

Hydrazine Sulfate

Hydrazine sulfate has been evaluated as a treatment for cancer-related anorexia and cachexia because of its ability to inhibit gluconeogenesis and in vitro data suggesting it inhibits tumor necrosis factor (TNF) cytolytic activity in cell cultures (19). Three large placebo-controlled trials of hydrazine sulfate for the treatment of cancer-related weight loss have failed to demonstrate either increased appetite or weight gain with hydrazine sulfate, as shown in Table 13.5.

Table 13.5   Placebo-Controlled Trials of Hydrazine Sulfate

Patient Population	Treatment	Appetite
Non-small cell lung cancer (20)	Chemotherapy and placebo or hydrazine sulfate	No improvement
Small cell lung cancer (21)	Chemotherapy and placebo or hydrazine sulfate	No improvement
Colorectal cancer (22)	Placebo or hydrazine sulfate	No improvement

Side Effects

No significant toxicity.

Conclusion

Although the treatment was well-tolerated, the lack of demonstrated benefit from hydrazine sulfate for the amelioration of cancer-associated anorexia across all three trials, dampens any enthusiasm for its recommendation or further evaluation.

Anabolic Agents

Anabolic agents, a potential intervention for cancer-associated cachexia, have not been well-evaluated. While a number of agents (growth hormone, oxandrolone, nandrolone) are either approved or currently being evaluated for the treatment of AIDS-associated weight loss, little data is available regarding their use in cancer-associated cachexia.

Metoclopramide

Early satiety as a result of delayed gastric emptying and gastroparesis may occur in up to 60% of patients with anorexia and cancer-related weight loss (23). Metoclopramide, an antiemetic and prokinetic agent, may relieve cancer-related anorexia, particularly when associated with dysmotility. In a small phase II study in advanced cancer patients with anorexia, metoclopramide, 10 mg QID, improved anorexia in 17 of 20 patients (24).

Side Effects

Diarrhea occurs infrequently at this dose. Hyperactivity is common and responds to dose reduction.

Conclusion

Delayed gastric emptying is common in patients with advanced cancer and may be exacerbated by the decrease in gut motility associated with narcotic analgesic use. This agent should be considered for any patient who complains of early satiety and anorexia.

Summary

The medical management of anorexia and cachexia requires a careful evaluation of symptoms and medications that may interfere with adequate intake. If specific, easily reversible symptoms (ie, nausea, mucositis) cannot be identified then pharmacologic agents should be considered. An intervention should be chosen based on the patient's treatment goals and his/her prognosis. For patients with very limited survival, (< 3 months) whose primary goal is to increase the enjoyment of eating, megestrol acetate or corticosteroids may be useful. For the majority of patients, treatment is intended to improve oral intake, weight, and, ideally, function. To achieve this, an approach which combines an appetite-enhancing agent (ie, dronabinol, megestrol acetate, corticosteroids, metoclopramide) with exercise and an anabolic medication may be ideal (see section on "Anabolic Agents"). For additional information on medications used for oncology treatment, see Chapter 6, *Chemotherapy and Nutrition Implications,* and Appendix B, *Common Supportive Drug Therapies.*

References

1. Sallan SE, Cronin C, Zelan M, Zinberg NE. Antiemetics in patients receiving chemotherapy for cancer: A randomized comparison of delta-9-tetrahydrocannabinol and prochlorperazine. *N Engl J Med.* 1976;302:135-138.

2. Wadleigh R, Spaulding M, Lembersky B, et al. Dronabinol enhancement of appetite in cancer patients [abstract]. *Am Soc Clin Oncol.* 1990;9:331.

3. Nelson K, Walsh D, Deeter P, Sheehan F. A phase II study of delta-9-tetrahydrocannabinol for appetite stimulation in cancer-associated anorexia. *J Palliat Care.* 1994;10:14-18.

4. Gorter R, Seefrid M, Volberding P. Dronabinol effects on weight in patients with HIV infection. *AIDS.* 1992;6:127-128.

5. Beal JE, Olson R, Laubernstein L, et al. Dronabinol as a treatment for anorexia associated with weight loss in patients with AIDS. *J Pain Symptom Management.* 1995;2:89-97.

6. Gregory EJ, Cohen SC, Oives DW. Megestrol acetate therapy for advanced breast cancer. *J Clin Oncol.* 1985;3:155-160.

7. Tchekmedyian NS, Tait A, Mandy M, Aisner J. High dose megestrol acetate: a possible treatment for cachexia. *JAMA.* 1987;9:1195-1198.

8. Loprinzi CL, Ellison NM, Schaid DJ, Krook JE, Athmann LU, Dose AM, Mailliard JA, Johnson PA, Ebbert LP, Geeraerts LA. Controlled trial of megestrol acetate for the treatment of cancer anorexia and cachexia. *J Natl Cancer Inst.* 1990;82:1127-1132.

9. Bruera E, MacMillan K, Kuehn N, Hanson J, MacDonald RN. A controlled trial of megestrol acetate on appetite, calorie intake, nutritional status and other symptoms in patients with advanced cancer. *Cancer.* 1990;66:1279-1282.

10. Tchekmedyian NS, Tait N, Moody M, Greco FA, Aisner J. Appetite stimulation with megestrol acetate in cachectic cancer patients. *Semin Oncol.* 1986;13:37-43.

11. Moertel C, Schulte A, Reitemeier R. Corticosteroid therapy of preterminal gastrointestinal cancer. *Cancer.* 1974;33:1607-1609.

12. Wilcox J, Corr J, Shaw J. Prednisone as an appetite stimulant in patients with cancer. *Br Med J.* 1984;200:37.

13. Bruera E, Roca E, Cedaro L, Carraros, Chacon R. Action of oral methylprednisolone in terminal cancer patients: a prospective randomized double-blind study. *Cancer Treat Rep.* 1985;69:751-754.

14. Robustelli Della Cuna G, Pellegrini A, Piazzi M. Effect of methylprednisolone sodium succinate on quality of life in pre-terminal cancer patients: A placebo controlled, multi-center study. *Eur J Cancer Clin Oncol.* 1989;25:1817-1821.

15. Popiela T, Lucchi R, Giongo F. Methylprednisolone as palliative therapy for female terminal cancer patients. *Eur J Cancer Clin Oncol.* 1989;25:1923-1929.

16. Loprinzi CL, Kugler J, Slvon J, Maillaid J, Krook J, Wilwerding M, Rowland K. Phase II randomized comparison of megestrol acetate, dexamethasone and fluoxymesterone for the treatment of cancer anorexia/cachexia [abstract]. *Proc Amer Soc Clin Oncol.* 1997;167.

17. Kardinal C, Loprinzi C, Shaid DS, Hags AC, Dose AM, Athmann LM, Mailliard JA, McCormack GW, Gerstner JB, Schray MF. A controlled trial of cyproheptadine in cancer patients with anorexia. *Cancer.* 1980;65:2657-2662.

18. Summerbell CD, Youle M, McDonald V, Catalan J, Gazzard BG. Megestrol acetate versus cyproheptadine in the treatment of weight loss associated with HIV infection. *Intl J of STD and AIDS.* 1992;3:278-280.

19. Hughes TK, Cadet P, Larned CS. Modulation of tumor necrosis factor activities by a potential anti-cachexia compound, hydrazine sulfate. *Int J Immunopharmacol.* 1989;11:501-507.

20. Kosty MP, Fleishman SB, Hendon JE II, Coughlin K, Kornblith AB, Scalzo A, Morris JC, Mortimer J, Green MR. Cisplatin, vinblastine and hydrazine sulfate in advanced non-small cell lung cancer: a randomized placebo-controlled double blind phase III study of the cancer and leukemia group. *Br J Clin Oncol.* 1994;12:1113-1120.

21. Loprinzi CL, Goldberg RM, Su JQ, Maillard JA, Kuross SA, Maksymiute AW, Kugler JW, Jett JR, Ghosh C, Pfeifle DNl. Placebo-controlled trial of hydrazine sulfate in patients with newly diagnosed non-small cell lung cancer. *J Clin Oncol.* 1994;12:1126-1129.

22. Loprinzi CL, Kuross SA, O'Fallon JR, Gesme DH Jr, Gerstner JB, Rospha RN, Cobau CD, Goldbert RM. Randomized placebo-controlled evaluation of hydrazine sulfate in patients with advanced colorectal cancer. *J Clin Oncol.* 1994;12(6):1121–1125.

23. Curtis EB, Krech R, Walsh TD. Common symptoms in patients with advanced cancer. *J Palliat Care.* 1991;7:25–29.

24. Kris MG, Yeh SDJ, Gralla RJ. Symptomatic gastroparesis in cancer patients—a possible cause of cancer-associated anorexia that can be improved with oral metoclopramide [abstract]. *Proc Am Soc Clin Oncol.* 1985;4:1038A.

Suggested Reading

Bruera E. Is the pharmacologic treatment of cancer cachexia possible? *Supportive Care in Cancer.* Nov 1993;1(6):298–304.

Nelson KA, Walsh D, Sheehn FA. The cancer anorexia-cachexia syndrome. *J Clin Oncol.* 1994;12(1):213–225.

Ottery FD, Walsh D, Strawford A. Pharmacologic management of anorexia/cachexia. *Semin in Oncol.* 1998;26(suppl 6):35–44.

14

Medical Nutrition Therapy in HIV Disease

Cade Fields-Gardner, MS, RD

Because the immunocompromised patient is at higher risk for neoplasm, the oncology specialist is likely to see patients with HIV disease in his or her practice. This chapter will discuss the issues facing patients with HIV disease and their care providers.

The "Face of AIDS" is rapidly changing. Since the observation of immune deficiency and discovery of the human immunodeficiency virus (HIV) as the etiologic agent of the acquired immunodeficiency syndrome (AIDS) in the early 1980s, much has been learned about retroviruses, immune deficiency, and opportunistic infections. Though not initially recognized by many HIV-specialist clinicians and researchers, nutrition-related issues play a primary role in the process, progress, and treatment of HIV disease (1-3).

Natural History of HIV Disease

Once HIV infects the body, a typical viral process ensues. Unlike many other viruses, it appears that there is no "dormant phase" (4). The virus seems to settle into an equilibrium where the numbers generated in the host cells (CD4 cells that orchestrate the immune system functions) are enough to replace the lost virus and maintain a static "viral load" or "viral burden." Research suggests that the higher the viral equilibrium or "set point," the quicker immune dysfunction occurs and disease progresses. Therefore, the primary goal of therapy is to reduce and even eliminate evidence of viral presence to prevent, halt, and perhaps even reverse immunologic damage that can lead to disease progression (5). Disease progression that occurs with decreases in CD4 count and/or increases in viral load affects the body's ability to maintain a favorable nutrition status.

Nutrition Issues in HIV Disease

Though the ability to control HIV is of primary concern, the reduction of viral load does not appear to automatically reverse existing malnutrition (6). Food and nutrient interactions with the antiretroviral medications are common and many times it is difficult for patients to cope with the complexities of medication adherence (7,8). Improvements in nutrition status, and particularly in lean body mass, are significantly associated with clinical well-being (improvement and stability of clinical markers such as laboratory values) and quality of life despite the level of HIV in the blood (9,10). Maintenance of optimal nutrition status is essential not only to the integrity of the body's stores, but also to the support of medications and other therapies used to combat disease.

Nutrition and immune function are intertwined. Therefore, any compromise in nutrition status can contribute to HIV disease progression. Nutrition status may be compromised by HIV and its related complications in several ways. These issues may be categorized as either nutrient inadequacy or altered nutrient metabolism (11). During primary infections, the body undergoes a normal stress response as the immune system is activated to protect the body. This stress response may or may not represent the first assault on nutrition status. In many cases, predisposition to or pre-existing malnutrition may undermine a normal immune response. Hypermetabolism and preferential loss of the body's lean tissue are hallmarks of stress responses. The chronic inflammation caused by HIV infection makes the stress response a continuous and mostly unrelenting process.

The stress response is also marked by loss of appetite and reduced nutrient intake. Specific risk factors for diminished nutrient intake include anorexia, nausea/vomiting, diarrhea or constipation, or inadequate food security (including availability, economic resources, transportation, and other details tied to the person's ability to secure adequate food supplies). Complicating factors include alteration in gastrointestinal and related functions that lead to malabsorption. Malabsorption, especially of fat-based substances, may be caused by injury to gastrointestinal cells, lymphatic blocks, altered motility, long-term antibiotic therapies, exocrine pancreatic dysfunction, and intestinal neuropathy among other complications (12).

The body's response to the viral infection may alter nutrient storage and function. Hypermetabolism of energy and shunting of acute phase reactant nutrients and molecules, such as iron and albumin as seen in infection and injury, may be perpetual in HIV disease. Endocrine dysfunction, such as insulin resistance, hypogonadism, and endogenous growth hormone resistance, may further contribute to altered use of nutrient stores such as micronutrients, skeletal muscle, and lipid deposition (13). Cellular antioxidant supplies may be depleted with oxidative stress and contribute to the immune dysfunction and cellular destruction that occurs with HIV infection (14).

Nutrition Assessment
Diet History

Evaluation of the person infected with HIV is similar to that of other patients. It appears that the primary factor associated with weight loss is decreased nutrient intake (15,16). Therefore, a diet history is an important part of an initial and follow-up assessment. Comparisons of actual intake with estimated needs should be made for each patient. Estimations of safe and adequate intake of macro- and micronutrients are currently based on typical calculations used in other disease states. Equations such as Harris-Benedict for energy needs and high protein levels (150 calories:1 gram nitrogen) for protein rehabilitation can be used depending on individual tolerance (17,18).

Medical History

An additional factor to consider is the history and degree of immune dysfunction and resulting complications. Opportunistic infections and neoplasms present additional challenges to nutrition well-being by exacerbating the stress response.

Nutrition-related symptoms such as anorexia, nausea, vomiting, diarrhea, and others that accompany HIV infection, opportunistic infections, and antibiotic therapies may interfere with adequate nutrient intake. Nutrition evaluation and intervention should also be tailored for conditions not associated with HIV infection, including altered organ function (renal, hepatic, pancreatic, pulmonary, cardiovascular, gonadal, and others) (19). Information on organ function can help to assess the patient's ability to maintain nutrition status (eg., gonadal function is assessed to determine the ability to produce testosterone and maintain muscle mass and prevent anemia).

Biochemical Assessment

Because HIV disease is a chronic inflammatory disease, it is difficult to interpret many laboratory values that may be used as markers of nutrition status (20). What is "normal" for HIV+ persons is unknown, but likely to be a heterogeneous profile (21). For instance, a drop in serum albumin may represent the processes associated with infection or injury more so than a change in nutrition status (19). Iron stores may be shunted into storage forms as seen in anemias of chronic disease (19). As needed, functional laboratory analysis (tests that relate nutrition status to the performance of organs and cells) has been recommended to augment the more readily available blood work such as albumin or even more labor intensive, creatinine-height index and nitrogen balance (19).

Other clues of malnutrition are hormonal levels and function. For example, decreased testosterone levels reduce ability to maintain muscle stores and present a risk factor for anemia (22,23). However, an understanding and consensus as to whether or not alterations in hormonal levels are a "normal" response or a protective mechanism in HIV disease remains elusive.

Physical Assessment

Physical assessment of body integrity and changes can offer information on nutrition status (24) and individual responses to HIV and its treatment. An overview may include evidence of wasting or alterations in body shape (19). Temporal wasting and the loss of facial fat pads appear in some patients. Thinning extremities and enlarged bellies or lipid deposits in the dorsocervical area appear in some (dubbed the "lipodystrophy syndrome"). While our first response is to correct undesirable alterations, nutrition and exercise may be only part of the solution. Researchers continue to be confounded by such changes, and no consensus on cause or solution is available at this time (25,26).

Anthropometry including midarm, waist and thigh circumferences; triceps, biceps, subscapular, suprailiac, abdominal, and thigh fatfolds; and body composition analysis through bioelectrical impedance analysis, dual x-ray absorptiometry, deuterium oxide, and/or total body postassium evaluations can further define protein, fluid, and fat stores and help the clinician determine the nature of weight loss, gain, and maintenance (19). Additional physical assessment, including a review of skin, hair, eyes, oral cavity, and other characteristics, along with dietary, medical, and medication histories can provide clues about nutrient deficiencies or toxicities.

Interventions

Malnutrition and wasting is a heterogeneous process in HIV disease (20,21,27). The process is likely to include combinations of risk factors that are either unique to HIV disease or common in other chronic diseases. Successful intervention aimed at preservation, rehabilitation, and enhancement of nutrition status is likely to be a result of an individually tailored set of combination therapies. These therapies may be categorized into (1) nutrition support; (2) activity and exercise; (3) treatment for HIV and immune restoration; (4) prevention and prompt, effective treatment of opportunistic infections and/or neoplasms; and (5) control of undesirable symptoms or side effects of HIV disease and its treatment (including inflammatory and hormonal modulation) (28). Nutrition support may include diet education, medical nutrition supplementation, enteral delivery of nutrients, and/or parenteral nutrition. Activity and exercise are tailored to the client's ability and need, usually consisting of some form of aerobic and resistance activity to build endurance and body cell mass. Appropriate treatment for HIV disease and infection or neoplastic complications may involve early diagnosis, medications, and other treatments that are matched to the client's needs. Symptoms are controlled through medication and other strategies, such as dietary alterations to reduce diarrhea.

Each of the intervention categories of treatment are interdependent. Antiretroviral therapies are greatly dependent on reaching a therapeutic level in the blood which requires close attention to the presence and timing of food and types of macronutrients in the diet (see Table 14.1). Activity and exercise are dependent on available nutrient substrate, including macro- and micronutrients, and hormonal balance, such as the level and response of the body to insulin, sex hormones, cortisol, growth homone, and others that regulate body composition and function. Adequate and effective treatment for complicating infections are dependent on the body's fluid, protein, and micronutrient storage and function. Unwanted symptoms and side effects, such as anorexia, nausea, vomiting, diarrhea, bloating, reflux, and pain, can limit the body's tolerance to medications, nutrition support, and antiretroviral therapies.

Table 14.1 Manufacturers' Information on Selected Antiretroviral Medication and Food Interactions

Generic Name	Brand Name/Company	Without Food	Without Regard to Food	With Food	With Nonfat Food	With High-Fat Food
Abacavir	Ziagen/Glaxo-SmithKline, Research Triangle Park, NC		x			
Adefovir	Preveon/Gilead, Foster City, CA		x[1]			
Amprenavir	Agenerase/Glaxo-SmithKline, Research Triangle Park, NC		x			
Delaveridine mesylate	Rescriptor/Pharmacia and Upjohn, Kalamazoo, MI		x[2]			
Didanosine (ddI)	Videx/Bristol-Myers Squibb, Princeton, NJ	x[3]				
Efavirenz	Sustiva/DuPont, Wilmington, DE		x			
Hydroxyurea	Hydrea/Bristol-Myers Squibb, Princeton, NJ Hydroxyurea/Roxane, Columbus, OH		x[4]			
Indinavir sulfate	Crixivan/Merck, West Point, PA	x[5]			x	
Lamivudine (3TC)	Epivir/Glaxo-SmithKline, Research Triangle Park, NC		x[6]			
Nelfinavir mesylate	Viracept/Agouron, La Jolla, CA			x[7]		
Nevirapine	Viramune/Roxane, Columbus, OH		x			
Ritonavir	Norvir/Abbott, Abbott Park, IL			x[8]		
Saquinavir mesylate	Invirase or Fortovase/Roche, Nutley, NJ			x[9]		x
Stavudine (d4T)	Zerit/Bristol-Myers Squibb, Princeton, NJ		x[10]			
Zalcitibine (ddC)	Hivid/Roche, Nutley, NJ	x[11]				
Zidovudine (AZT, ZVD)	Retrovir/Glaxo-SmithKline, Research Triangle Park, NC			x	x[12]	

[1]Daily 500 mg L-carnitine supplement is recommended to prevent significant carnitine deficiency
[2]Take 1 hour after or before didanosine; do not take with antacids
[3]Alcohol may exacerbate toxicity
[4]Assure adequate fluid intake
[5]Take on empty stomach 1 hour before or 2 hours after meals; drink plenty of fluids (8–10 cups/day); grapefruit juice may decrease absorption; use of indinavir in combination with ritonavir eliminates food restriction
[6]Though absorption is decreased with food, systemic availability was not affected
[7]Take with meal or light snack
[8]Take with foods that contain protein and fat; taste may need to be masked with food or beverages; place liquid in back of mouth to swallow (use straw)
[9]Take within 2 hours of full meal; high-fat, high-calorie meal improves systemic availability 2–7 times; grapefruit juice may increase absorption
[10]Though absorption is decreased with food, systemic availability was not affected; contains lactose
[11]Do not take with antacids
[12]High-fat meal may decrease peak plasma concentrations; take with low-fat or light meal

Nutrition Support

Provision of adequate nutrients is currently a "best guess" based on estimated needs. Maintenance level goals for fluid, calorie, protein, and micronutrient intake may be implemented and increased once tolerance for feeding is established (19). Overfeeding may be an additional concern, especially in patients with compromised lung and kidney function. Additional nutrients may be required for patients who appear to be using more or absorbing less. In some cases, long term medication therapy may require micronutrient or other types of nutrient supplementation. For example, the antiretroviral medication adefovir severely depletes the body's carnitine levels and requires 500 mg of oral L-carnitine supplementation to prevent life-threatening deficiency. Some practitioners have also employed experimental use of pharmacologic doses of macro- and micronutrients, such as fish oils, to reduce inflammatory proesses and antioxidant nutrients to help replenish intracellular supplies, to reduce effects of oxidative stress and enhance muscle and immune function (29). Though supplementation with at least a well-balanced multivitamin/mineral product is a common recommendation, controversy exists as to the actual value and function of supplemented nutrients in this population. There is no consensus or consistency in micronutrient recommendations for patients with HIV disease.

Nutrient-based therapies to enhance nutrient availability may include specialized diet, oral supplementation, enteral, and parenteral strategies. Examples are low-residue diets, medium-chain triglyceride-containing medical nutrition supplements, elemental enteral formulas, and glutamine-enriched parenteral nutrition. Tolerance to fats, protein, and carbohydrates may require dietary manipulation (28,30). Each of these approaches must consider all medical diagnoses, cultural issues, and other conditions that may affect the need for emphasis or restriction in an individual's diet.

Numerous side effects can be caused by disease, medications, and malnutrition. Symptom management strategies such as dietary manipulation, antidiarrheal and antiemetic medications may be essential to the tolerance and efficacy of medications and nutrition therapies. Symptom management can be used in conjunction with therapies aimed at overcoming medical complications.

Anorexia is a common complication of HIV infection, its complications, and its treatments. Psychosocial issues and infectious processes can also lead to loss of appetite. Dietary strategies in conjunction with appetite stimulant medication (eg., megestrol acetate or dronabinol) may help to prevent long-term problems of inadequate nutrient intake (see Chapter 13, *Pharmacological Management of Anorexia and Cachexia*).

Long-term antibiotic therapies may contribute to gastrointestinal symptoms and malabsorption. Antidiarrheal medications used along with prescription pancrelipase therapy may prove valuable in patients with pancreatic dysfunction to enhance nutrient absorption and diminish diarrhea, bloating, or other symptoms associated with malabsorption (31,32).

Adjunctive Therapies

Activity and resistance exercise become important therapies to maintain and enhance lean tissues, particularly the skeletal muscle tissues that are often preferentially lost in stress responses (33). Aerobic exercise to build endurance and additional exercise to improve flexibility are also recommended on a routine basis. Little research has been done in the arena of exercise in HIV disease, though two studies suggest an important role in maintaining and enhancing nutrition status to improve desired clinical outcomes, such as improved lean body mass, reduced infection rates, improved CD4 count, and enhanced quality of life (33,34).

Anticytokines work to block the protein-catabolizing effects of cytokine protein mediators during stress responses. In HIV disease, as in other chronic conditions, the continued, and sometimes inappropriate, production and presence of cytokine mediators may induce significant protein tissue wasting. Because inflammatory processes may play an important role in the precipitation of weight loss and wasting syndrome, anticytokine therapies (such as thalidomide) have been studied and demonstrate some lean tissue gain and clinical improvement (35).

Hormonal alterations may be a consequence of HIV disease, complications that affect organ function, medication interactions, and/or weight loss. Normalization or enhancement of hormonal level and function is the subject of much current research. Resistance to endogenous hormones may require medication therapies, such as insulin sensitizers and other therapies, such as exercise. Of particular interest is the therapeutic use for growth hormone and anabolic steroids (such as testosterone metabolites or synthetic versions in injectable, oral, nasal, sublingual, or patch forms). Short-term and intermittent use of these therapies has been studied. However, long-term use of anti-wasting therapies at physiologic or pharmacologic doses have yet to be studied for safety and continued efficacy.

Monitoring and Adjusting Therapies

As with all nutrition care plans, it is important to monitor patient status and adjust therapies as appropriate. Medical nutrition therapy protocols for use in HIV disease have been developed to address the process of assessment, intervention, and monitoring client nutrition status (36). Nutrition assessments are recommended according to the acuity of each individual's clinical status. For example, ongoing assessment every three to six months is appropriate in asymptomatic stages to update clinical information and educational needs.

During acute events, a client may need more constant, weekly or even daily monitoring. Chronic complicating factors, such as diabetes or renal insufficiency may require regular visits to stabilize clinical status. An important goal in providing education for the patient is to support self-care.

Infectious Disease Precautions

When an individual is immune compromised, it is important to protect against exposure to infectious disease. The dietetics profession can provide input on food safety issues that may protect the patient from unnecessary risk of food-borne illness. Special attention should be paid to uncooked or undercooked fresh fruits, vegetables, and protein foods. Safe food procurement, storage, and handling are all important training topics for patients and health care providers.

In addition, care providers should use and provide education on "universal precautions" for the prevention of disease exposure (37). The primary concern for the clinician, other care providers, family, and friends is exposure to HIV and its complicating infectious disease. For details on universal precautions refer to the *Red Cross HIV Fact Book* or facility protocols (37).

Summary

Nutrition issues in HIV disease challenge clinical, community, and food service dietetics professionals in many ways. Clinical evaluation and intervention require knowledge of issues that confront the HIV-infected person. These issues may include immune compromise, organ dysfunction, and non–HIV-related health issues. Additional consideration is required for psychosocial and economic issues. Appropriate support from the dietetics professional includes compassion and absence of bias in developing supportive patient-oriented goals, objectives, and outcomes measurements.

Improvement of nutrition status may require more than nutrition support. Additional considerations include immune dysfunction, history of infection, endocrine function, symptoms and side effects, and physical limitations. As such, a team approach will be essential to fully addressing nutrition status preservation and rehabilitation in persons who are HIV-infected.

Glossary of Terms Relating to HIV Disease

AIDS Acquired immunodeficiency syndrome, the symptomatic manifestation of immune deficiency in persons who are infected with HIV

Anticytokine therapies Therapies such as thalidomide or other substances aimed at the reduction of cytokines (such as tumor necrosis factor or interleukins) that may initiate inflammatory and tissue wasting processes

CD4 cell A T-cell (type of immune cell) that orchestrates immune function

HIV Human immunodeficiency virus, the etiologic agent of AIDS

Inflammatory modulation Pharmacologic efforts to alter the process and/or impact of inflammation on body stores

Opportunistic infection An infection that occurs in immune insufficiency that would not occur in persons with adequately functioning immune systems

Primary infection Initial stage of infection that causes immune sensitivity to invading infectious cells; includes rise in white blood cell count

Retrovirus A virus that carries RNA that must be transcribed into DNA strands

Wasting syndrome CDC defines as >10% weight loss along with fever or diarrhea for more than 30 days of unknown origin; clinical definition is based on unintentional weight loss and lean tissue loss

Viral load The number of viral particles expressed as copies per milliliter of blood

References

1. American Dietetic Association (with Dietitians of Canada). Position of the American Dietetic Association. Nutrition intervention in the care of persons with human immunodeficiency virus infection. *J Am Diet Assoc.* 2000;100. In press.
2. Palenicek JP, Graham NMH, He YD, Hoover DA, Oishi JS, Kingsley L, Saah AJ. Weight loss prior to clinical AIDS as a predictor or survival. *J Acquir Imm Defic Syndr Hum Retrovir.* 1995;10(3):366–373.
3. Kotler DP, Tierney AR, Wang J, Pierson RN. Magnitude of body-cell-mass depletion and the timing of death from wasting in AIDS. *Am J Clin Nutr.* 1989;50:444–447.
4. Ho DD. Viral counts count in HIV infection. *Science.* 1996;272:1124–1125.
5. Bartlett JG. *Pocket Book of Infectious Disease Therapy.* 8th ed. Baltimore, Md: Williams & Wilkins; 1997.
6. Teixeira A, Leu JC, Honderlick P, Trylesinski A, Zucman D. Variation in body weight and plasma viral load in HIV patients treated with therapy including a protease inhibitor [abstract]. *Nutrition.* 1997;13(3):269.
7. Pronsky Z. *Food-Medication Interactions.* 10th ed. Pottstown, Pa: Food-Medication Interactions; 1997.
8. Pronsky Z, Fields-Gardner C. *Food-Medication Interactions in HIV/AIDS.* Pottstown, Pa: Food-Medication Interactions; 1998.
9. Sharpstone D, Ross M, Murray C, Phelaw M, Gazzard B. The influence of nutrition and metabolic status on progression from asymptomatic HIV infection to AIDS [abstract]. *Nutrition.* 1997;13(3):270.
10. McKinley MJ, Goodman-Lock J, Salbe AD. Improved nutrition status as a result of nutrition intervention in adult HIV outpatients [abstract]. IX Int'l Conf on AIDS. 1993;9(1):529.
11. Hellerstein MK, Kahn J, Mudie H, Viteri F. Current approach to the treatment of human immunodeficiency virus-associated weight loss: pathophysiologic considerations and emerging management strategies. *Semin Oncol.* 1990;17(6 suppl 9):17–33.
12. Tanowitz H, Simon D, Wittner M. Gastrointestinal manifestations of AIDS. *Med Clin North Am.* 1991;76:45S–62S.
13. Coodley GO, Loveless MO, Nelson HD, Coodley MK. Endocrine function in the HIV wasting syndrome. *J AIDS.* 1994;7(1):46–51.
14. Lalonde RG, McDermid JM, Kubow S, Gray-Donald K. Diet and supplements do not reduce oxidative stress in clinically stable persons with HIV infection [abstract]. XI Int'l Conf on AIDS. 1996;11(2):101.
15. Macallan DC, Noble C, Baldwin C, Foskett M, McManus T, Griffin GE. Prospective analysis of patterns of weight change in stage IV human immunodeficiency virus infection. *Am J Clin Nutr.* 1993;58:417–424.
16. Grunfeld C, Pang M, Shimizu L, Shigenaga JK, Jensen P, Feingold KK. Resting energy expenditure, caloric intake and short-term weight change in human immunodeficiency virus infection and the acquired immunodeficiency syndrome. *Am J Clin Nutr.* 1992;55:455–460.
17. Macallan DC, Noble C, Baldwin C, Jebb SA, Prentice AM, Coward WA, Sawyer MB, McManus TJ, Griffin GE. Energy expenditure and wasting in human immunodeficiency virus infection. *N Eng J Med.* 1995;333(2):83–88.
18. Bowers JM, Ampel NM, Scott RW, Dols CL, Campbell S. Indirect calorimetry in HIV-infected patients [abstract]. XI Int'l Conf on AIDS. 1996;11(2):102.
19. Fields-Gardner C, Thomson CA, Rhodes SS. *A Clinician's Guide to Nutrition in HIV and AIDS.* Chicago, IL: American Dietetic Association; 1997.
20. Hellerstein MK, Neese R, Papageorgopoulos C, Hoh R. Multiple abnormalities in lipid and carbohydrate metabolism in men with AIDS-wasting syndrome (AWS) inter-individual variability, pathophysiologic mechanisms and prognostic significance [abstract]. XI Int'l Conf on AIDS. 1996;11(1):332–333.
21. Hoh R, Strawford A, Hellerstein MK. Spontaneous changes in body composition, hormonal, and metabolic parameters in AIDS patients followed longitudinally [abstract]. XI Int'l Conf on AIDS. 1996;11(1):124.
22. Engelson ES, Goggin KJ, Rabkin JG, Kotler DP. Nutrition and testosterone status of HIV+ women [abstract]. XI Int'l Conf on AIDS. 1996;11(1):332.
23. Sattler FR, Antonipaillai I, Allen J, Briggs W, Horton R. Wasting and sex hormones: evidence for the pathogenesis of dihydrotestosterone in AIDS patients from weight loss [abstract]. XI Int'l Conf on

AIDS. 1996;11(1):331.

24. Kight MA. The nutrition physical examination. *CRN Quart*. 1987;11(3):9-12.

25. Batterham M. Lipodystrophy—a side effect of protease inhibitor therapy. *Pos Commun*. 1998;2(2):1-5.

26. Fields-Gardner C. Interview of four physicians on lipodystrophy. *Pos Commun*. 1998;2(3):4-6.

27. Hellerstein MK. Pathophysiology of lean body mass wasting and nutrient unresponsiveness in HIV/AIDS: therapeutic implications. In: *Proceedings of 1992 Int'l Conf on Nutr and HIV/AIDS*. Chicago, IL: PAAC;1993:17-25.

28. Cohan GR, Fields-Gardner C. Malnutrition and wasting in HIV disease: a review. *Persp Appl Nutr*. 1994;2:10-19.

29. McDermid JM, Lalonde RG, Kubow S, Gray-Donald K. Elevated energy intake and antioxidant supplementation practices in clinically stable persons with HIV infection [abstract]. XI Int'l Conf on AIDS. 1996;11(2):101.

30. Koch J, Scott MK, Steuerwald MH, Keiserman M, Garcia-Shelton YL, Cello JP. Steatorrhea is nearly universal in patients with HIV-associated unexplained weight loss or diarrhea [abstract]. *Nutrition*. 1997;13(3):268.

31. Fields-Gardner C, Berger DS, Gocke M, Dieterich D, Capozza C. Clinical effects and nutrition benefits of pancreatic enzyme therapy in HIV+ patients with chronic diarrhea. Abstract presented at the ANAC Conference, Ft. Lauderdale, FL, November 1997.

32. Razecca K, Odenheimer S, Davis M, Landeck K. The treatment of nelfinavir induced diarrhea [abstract]. 12th World AIDS Conference. 1998;12:90.

33. Roubenoff R, Suri J, Raymond J, Fauntleroy J, Gorbach S. Feasibility of increasing lean body mass in HIV-infected adults using progressive resistance training [abstract]. *Nutrition*. 1997;13(3):271.

34. MacArthur RD, Levin SD, Birk TJ. Cardiopulmonary, immunologic and psychologic responses to exercise training in individuals seropositive for HIV. (PuB7327) VIII Int Conf on AIDS. 1192;8:103.

35. Reyes-Teran G, Sierra-Madero JG, Martinez del Cerro V, Arroyo-Figueroa H, Pasquetti A, Calva JJ, Ruiz-Palacios GM. Effects of thalidomide on HIV-associated wasting syndrome: a randomized, double-blind, placebo-controlled clinical trial. *AIDS*. 1996;10(13):1501-1507.

36. Gilbreath J, Inman-Felton AE, Johnson EQ, Robinson G, Smith KG (eds). *Medical Nutrition Therapy Across the Continuum of Care—Client Protocols*. 2nd ed. Chicago, Ill: The American Dietetic Association; 1998.

37. American Red Cross. Essential Facts About HIV and AIDS. In: HIV/AIDS Fact Book. Stock #32967. 1995:37-39.

Additional Resources

Professional Materials

Abdale F. *Community-Based Nutrition Support for People Living with HIV and AIDS: Technical Manual*. New York, NY: God's Love We Deliver; 1995. Contact GLWD at 212-274-1091.

Clum N. *Take Control: Living with HIV and AIDS*. Los Angeles, CA: AIDS Project Los Angeles; 1996. Contact APLA at 213-993-1600.

Fields-Gardner C, Thomson CA, Rhodes SS. *A Clinician's Guide to Nutrition in HIV and AIDS*. Chicago, IL: ADA; 1997.

Positive Communication. Quarterly newsletter of the HIV/AIDS Dietetic Practice Group of The American Dietetic Association.

Pronsky Z, Fields-Gardner C. *Food-Medication Interactions in HIV/AIDS*. Pottstown, PA: Food-Medication Interactions, Inc; 1998.

Client-Oriented Materials

Romeyn M. *Nutrition and HIV: A New Model for Treatment*. 2nd ed. San Francisco, CA: Jossey-Bass Publishers; 1997. ISBN# 0-7879-0107-5

McMillan L, Jarvie J, Brauer J. *Positive Cooking: Cooking for People Living with HIV*. Garden City Park, NY:

Avery Publishing Group; 1997. ISBN# 0-89529-734-5

Lehman RH. *Cooking for Life: A Guide to Nutrition and Food Safety for the HIV-Positive Community.* New York, NY: Dell Publishing; 1997.

Health Resources & Services Administration. *Health Care and HIV: Nutrition Guide for Providers and Clients.* Rockville, MD: HRSA Bureau of Primary Health Care; 1996. Contact Nutrition and HIV Manual at 703-442-9824.

National AIDS Manual: Nutrition. Pamphlet for patients written and published by NAM Publications, 16a Clapham Common Southside, London, England SW4 7AB; single copies may be obtained by calling 0171/627-3200; faxing 0171/627-3101; or email request to: admin@nam.org.uk.

American Red Cross. *HIV/AIDS Fact Book.* Stock #32967. 1995. Contact local American Red Cross Office.

Internet Sites

http://www.cdc.gov/nchstp/hiv_aids/dhap.htm
> Centers for Disease Control in Atlanta site with information in HIV infection, transmission, issues surrounding HIV disease, and treatment information.

http://www.hivatis.org/glossary
> Glossary of HIV/AIDS terms. Has HIV-related definitions and medication names.

http://www.eatright.org/nfs42.html
> Nutrition strategies for HIV/AIDS patients through ADA.

http://www.healthcg.com/hiv/treatment/interactions
> Information on this site includes updates from national and international meetings as well as reproduced guidelines from HIV publications. This subset of the site includes information on interactions with medications.

http://www.actis.org
> Information on recent treatment advances.

http://hivinsite.ucsf.edu/topics/research_advances/2098.339b.html
> Treatment information that includes medication interactions.

http://www.jag.on.ca/hiv/
> Medication interactions including food and nutrient interactions. Includes dietary suggestions on most drugs and drug-drug interactions with recommendations. Patient instructions and suggestions are printable for patient education. Read only Access (Microsoft) database in included to record and track patient data and generate medication schedules that include meal times and suggestions. Downloadable file (HIV Medication Guide) for use on individual computers is free (supported by a grant from Glaxo-Wellcome).

15

Medical Nutrition Therapy in Palliative Care

Anne Cox, MS, RD   Paula Davis McCallum, MS, RD

According to American Cancer Society Surveillance Search, the estimated number of cancer deaths for 1999 in the United States was 563,100 (1). Palliative care is defined as the active total care of a patient when curative measures are no longer considered an option by either the medical team or the patient. It is as aggressive as curative care, abolishing the philosophy that nothing more can be done. Palliative care is appropriate for any serious or life-threatening illness—even early in the course of disease when patients undergo active therapy or later, when they might be left with treatment-related morbidity that is ineffectively managed (2). The goal is optimal quality of life for patients and families through use of a multidisciplinary team approach to manage physiological symptoms such as pain, anorexia, nausea, and constipation, as well as psychological, social, and spiritual issues.

The term "hospice" refers to a concept of care. Palliative care is the approach used in hospice care. A Hospice Program can service patients in their homes, a residential hospice, nursing homes, adult foster care, or in the hospital. Medicare and insurance eligibility criteria for hospice care typically include a doctor's prognosis of "a life expectancy of six months or less." Studies show wide variation between such a prediction and actual survival; palliative care can be provided for years, if needed (3).

Goals of Nutrition Therapy in Palliative Medicine

Nutrition intervention focuses on managing symptoms of the disease or side effects of treatment, implementing appropriate medical nutrition therapy (MNT) to prevent further morbidity and to maintain optimal quality of life, and, when possible, providing sufficient dietary intake to maintain energy and strength (2,4,5,6).

Symptoms in Advanced Cancer

This chapter focuses on palliative care in patients with advanced, metastatic cancer who are no longer pursuing curative treatment. The most common nutrition-related symptoms in advanced cancer are listed in Table 15.1.

Table 15.1   Prevalence of Nutrition-Related Symptoms in Advanced Cancer

Symptom	Prevalence (n = 1000)
Pain	67%
Weakness	47%
Anorexia	46%
Weight loss	44%
Early satiety	33%
Constipation	31%
Dyspnea	28%
Dry mouth	27%
Depression	21%
Nausea	16%
Vomiting	10%
Taste changes	13%
Dysphagia	5%
Bloating	6%
Belching	6%
Diarrhea	2.5%
Hiccough	2%

Note: This data is taken from a prospective systematic analysis performed on 1000 consecutive consultations from 1990 to 1992 by the Palliative Care Service of the Cleveland Clinic Foundation (Ohio). The distribution of cancer diagnoses paralleled national statistics; diagnoses included lung, breast, colorectal, prostate, pancreas, kidney, head and neck, esophageal, gynecological, and unknown primary (7).

Pressure sores, dehydration, anemia, and hypercalcemia are also common and worthy of mention (6). It is important to be aware of the interrelationships among symptoms as exemplified in Box 15.1:

Box 15.1   Examples of Symptom Interrelationships (2,4,6,7,8)

Pain → Nausea → Anorexia → Weight loss → Cachexia

Constipation → Early satiety, nausea and/or vomiting → Weight loss → Cachexia

Stomatitis and/or oral candidasis → Dysphagia → Weight loss and/or dehydration → Constipation

Anxiety → Dyspnea → Air swallowing → Belching and/or bloating → Anorexia → Weight loss → Cachexia

Nausea → Vomiting → Dehydration and/or weight loss

Depression → Anorexia → Weight loss → Weakness

Radiation enteritis, malabsorption and/or lactose intolerance → Diarrhea → Dehydration and/or Weight loss

Anemia → Weakness → Inactivity → Pressure sores → Pain → Anorexia

Often alleviation of one symptom will resolve several others. Disease progression and medications can contribute significantly to patient symptoms (2,6). Wasting and decreased serum albumin may increase medication side effects and toxicity.

Management of Symptoms

Symptom management is covered in Appendix A. The following additional information should be considered in advanced disease (2,4,6,8–10):

Weight Loss Repletion of nutrition stores and regaining lost weight may not be reasonable goals. Note that people perceive weight loss differently and they should be treated accordingly . Use discretion in counseling so as not to diminish a patient's hope or will to live.

Hiccups Allow 15 to 30 minutes for hiccups to resolve on their own. Suggest taking a spoonful of sugar, followed by a full glass of water. Drinking one or more glasses of water while holding one's breath can also be helpful. To relieve gas, try peppermint or antacid. Medications such as metoclopramide or chlorpramazine may be effective.

Intestinal obstruction See following discussion of medical nutrition therapy.

Pressure sores Encourage adequate protein and calorie intake if possible to prevent further breakdown. Consider using a multivitamin with zinc and 500 mg vitamin C daily. Correct blood sugar elevations as much as possible.

Dehydration When death is not imminent, provide adequate hydration to maintain blood pressure, avoid electrolyte disturbance, combat constipation, and minimize nephrotoxic effects of medications. When death is imminent, dehydration is appropriate (see "Nutrition Intake When Death Is Imminent," page 141).

Anemia (iron-deficiency anemia) Prescribed iron supplements should be given with vitamin C to enhance absorption, and, at mealtime, to prevent gastritis. With poorer prognosis the side effects of constipation and nausea may outweigh the benefits.

Hypercalcemia Treat medically. Do not restrict calcium-containing foods; avoid calcium supplements or antacids.

Medical Nutrition Therapy

Maintenance of "Optimum Nutriture"

Maintenance of energy and strength is an appropriate goal that directly affects a patient's ability to perform activities of daily living. Oral intake can be enhanced with minor modifications of the patient's usual intake. See Appendix A, *Symptom Management for the Cancer Patient;* Chapter 4, *Calorie, Protein, Fluid, and Micronutrient Requirements;* and *Oncology Nutrition: Patient Education Materials,* a publication of the Oncology Nutrition Dietetic Practice Group of The American Dietetic Association (11).

Management of Alterations in Blood Glucose Levels

The goal in the patient with advanced cancer is to minimize symptoms associated with hypoglycemia or marked hyperglycemia. Patients generally feel better if blood sugars are controlled (8). Steroid-induced hyperglycemia is often temporary and usually requires minimal management unless polyuria and polydipsia warrant the need for an oral hypoglycemic agent (2). Weight loss and anorexia decrease the need for hypoglycemic agents as cancer progresses (2). Patients with type 1 diabetes have reduced requirements; simplification to a long-acting insulin injection once a day is appropriate. Dietary manipulation to control blood sugar must take into account patient desires, preferences, and ability to eat. Patients may prefer a simplified "no-added sugar" diet eaten at regular intervals if it can decrease the need for insulin (8). Patients with a longer life expectancy may prefer more intense dietary modifications to control blood sugar and prevent further morbidity.

Prevention of Bowel Obstruction

Etiology of intestinal obstruction in advanced cancer may be multifactorial. Causes include malignancy, motility disorders, inflammatory edema, fecal impaction, fibrosis, inelasticity and fatigue of the intestinal muscle, a change in fecal flora, and medications (2). Onset can be acute, or insidious and intermittent. Symptoms include abdominal pain and distention, anorexia and vomiting, and urinary incontinence. The degree of symptoms depends upon location of obstruction:

Duodenal obstruction: no pain, severe vomiting, no distention, and minimal bowel sounds
Small bowel obstruction: pain in upper to central abdomen, moderate to severe vomiting, moderate distention, and hyperactive bowel sounds with borborygmi
Large bowel obstruction: pain in the central to lower abdomen, subsequent vomiting, great distention, and borborygmi

Symptoms may resolve spontaneously. Patients can live an extended time period with intermittent partial obstruction. Treatment depends upon the cause, location, prognosis, condition, and patient wishes (6). Options include palliative surgery, gastrointestinal intubation for drainage, pharmacological administration (ie, steroids to decrease inflammation), and medical nutrition therapy. Usually, smooth muscle relaxants and analgesics, antiemetics, stool softeners, enemas, and suppositories are used to relieve symptoms (2,6,8).

Management

Allow patients to eat and drink if they wish; most prefer small frequent low- residue, mainly fluid meals. Patients may choose to avoid nausea or gas-precipitating foods, to sip fluids between meals, eat slowly, and eat their largest meal early in the day. Limiting high-fat foods is also helpful in reducing the incidence of early satiety. In some cases vomiting one to two times a day may be preferred to nasogastric tubes or suctioning. Adequate fluid and nutrients may be absorbed even with regular vomiting. High-potassium, high-calorie foods should be encouraged if this option is chosen. With complete obstruction, minimize oral intake (2,4,6).

Prevention

Prevent constipation with a regular bowel regimen and routine use of stool softeners/laxatives (refer to Appendix B, *Common Supportive Drug Therapies Used with Oncology Patients*); especially in patients with the greatest risk of developing obstruction, ie, post-abdominal surgery especially with radiation therapy, pancreatic, ovarian, colon cancer, and cases of abdominal carcinomatosis, mesenteric nodes, or metastases. Good prophylaxis of impending, intermittent, or partial obstruction can be achieved with a soft low-fiber diet void of raw fruits or vegetables, skins, nuts, seeds, or whole grains (11). Report symptoms regularly to the physician to ensure appropriate pharmacological management of constipation and intestinal motility.

Optimal Patient Comfort and Enjoyment (4,6,12,13)

- Provide favorite foods. Small frequent meals are often better tolerated.
- Use smaller plates and cups to make small portions look more complete and less overwhelming.
- Make eating area as attractive as possible; remove bedpans and other appliances that diminish appetite.
- Encourage patient to wash and dress for meals if possible.
- Encourage eating at table when possible.
- Encourage eating with others.
- Monitor patient likes and dislikes as tastes and preferences of the terminal patient can change frequently.
- Do not force food; remove food without incident if patient does not feel like eating.

- Maintain oral hygiene by rinsing patient's mouth with a baking soda mouthwash prior to eating.
- Encourage activity to stimulate appetite.
- Encourage patient to function as independently as possible to increase self-worth.
- Let the patient be in control.

Nutrient Requirements

Maintenance of physical and psychological strength for optimal quality of life is an appropriate goal (4). Nutrient requirements and determination of maintenance energy and protein needs are covered in Chapter 4, *Calorie, Protein, Fluid, and Micronutrient Requirements*. The following information applies to the terminal patient:

Energy Carbohydrates are usually well-tolerated and serve the purpose of sparing muscle and visceral protein, preventing ketosis, and supplying energy needs.

Protein Requirements for maintenance are appropriate unless diagnosis mandates restriction. High-protein diets do little to improve serum albumin level in this population (4,6).

Fat Fat, if tolerated, is a concentrated source of calories that can improve taste and texture of meals.

Fluid Encourage adequate hydration to alleviate constipation, dehydration, and drug toxicity. Determination of fluid needs is covered in Chapter 4, *Calorie, Protein, Fluid, and Micronutrient Requirements*.

Vitamin and Mineral Supplements Discontinue vitamin and mineral supplements that may contribute to GI distress, nausea, constipation, or diarrhea and therefore diminish quality of life (ie, iron supplements with severe constipation or nausea, potassium chloride with GI distress/difficulty swallowing).

Special Diets Special diets are only to be used to control symptoms and increase comfort. When restriction is necessary, tailor the diet according to individual preference. Use prudence in instructing patients to abandon diets that they may equate with longevity and hope; patients may prefer to stay on physician-ordered or unconventional diets. Modification of such diets can increase a patient's food selections and enjoyment while still upholding the basic dietary concepts (ie, low-salt, macrobiotic).

Nutrient Intake When Death is Imminent "A decrease in food and fluid intake at the end of life is normal and appears to be part of the natural physiology of dying"(14). In the last few weeks to days of life, there is decline in function of the upper and lower esophageal sphincters, accompanied by slowed peristalsis and decreased oral and hypopharyngeal sensation. The net effect is ketosis with significant anorexia, marked weight loss, energy loss, and fluid and electrolyte imbalance (6). Since maintenance of strength at this time is unrealistic, caregivers should be encouraged to show love and support in ways that do not involve food.

Dehydration

Terminal dehydration is "the clinical state of dying patients unable to consume adequate fluid volumes usually associated with maintenance hydration requirements" (15). Deprivation of water increases endogenous dynorphin, a very potent opiate (16). It also causes confusion and lethargy secondary to hyponatremia, which dulls the senses (17). The primary discomfort of dehydration is a dry mouth which can be alleviated with ice chips or moistened swabs (17). Cool fluids have been noted to be particularly satiating (14).

Artificial hydration at this time can decrease quality of life by its invasiveness and discomfort. Fluid overload from artificial hydration increases pulmonary and GI secretions, urinary output, and pharyngeal secretions that can potentiate the choking and gurgling sounds known as the "death rattle" (6). When a patient is receiving artificial hydration or nutrition support at the time of imminent death, it is appropriate to decrease amount of infusion to 500 to 600 mL per day to account for insensible fluid losses or to discontinue altogether if in accordance with patient and family desires (18).

Guidelines for the Use of Artificial Nutrition and Hydration in Palliative Care

Artificial Nutrition and Hydration (AN&H) is defined as "any nutrition and/or hydration support of an invasive nature requiring placement of a tube into the alimentary tract or parenterally via intravenous or subcutaneous means" (14).

According to the American Medical Association Code of Ethics, human dignity is the primary obligation when it conflicts with prolonging life. Court rulings over the last twenty years have established that all competent Americans have a constitutional right to accept or reject any or all medical treatment after comparing the risks and benefits. Refusal of such treatment is not suicide if the patient dies from the underlying disease/disorder (2,14,19–21).

In determining whether or not to initiate or discontinue nutrition support consider the following:

- Identify patient wishes. An advance directive identifying a patient's wishes with regard to AN&H is recommended to confirm patient desires and assist with decision making. The two most common forms are living wills and durable powers of attorney for health care. Patients are frequently asked to complete an advance directive upon admission to a nursing home, hospital, or hospice. A living will is a legal document specifying the kind of health care a patient does or does not desire. A durable power of attorney is a legal document wherein another person is given the authority to make medical decisions for the patient if he/she is unable. Advance directives can be changed or cancelled at any time according to respective state law. Even without written change, wishes expressed in person directly to the physician have more value than an advance directive if the patient is capable of making such decisions, and can communicate these wishes clearly (22,23). It is the medical team's responsibility to educate both the patient and caregivers on the benefits and burdens of AN&H so they can make an informed decision. *In the absence of an advance directive* patient wishes need to be clarified via either the patient, family member, or friend who is considered a reliable spokesperson. Individual states may require a "clear and convincing" evidence standard for patients without an advanced directive (13,22).

- Use patient autonomy as a guiding ethical principle (4,20,23,24). It is important to remember that pain, discomfort, and mental conditions such as depression, dementia, or delirium affect the ability to make rational decisions, and every effort should be made to stabilize a patient before such decisions are made (20).

- Remember that AN&H is considered life-sustaining medical therapy that is no different from drug therapy, surgery, dialysis, mechanical ventilation or any other medical interventions (14,23,24). Withholding or withdrawing AN&H holds the same ethical and legal significance: if a treatment is beneficial it is justified; if it ceases to be beneficial, it ceases to be justified. If the goal to maintain or improve strength is not realistic, nutrition support can ethically be discontinued with patient consent (4,6,23,24).

- Use AN&H to prolong life in accordance with a specifically defined goal and not for the sole purpose of delaying death. Use is appropriate in the following situations:
  1) A patient will succumb from malnutrition before succumbing to the primary diagnosis, eg, advanced dysphagia secondary to esophageal cancer (4,14).
  2) There is a need to resolve psychosocial issues, ie, business affairs, reconciliation, desire to attend a family event.
  3) A new, acute, curable diagnosis develops (eg, incidence of urosepsis in a patient with end-stage Alzheimer's), or a surgical procedure is needed for symptom control (eg, bowel obstruction in a patient with colon cancer) (2,14).

- Evaluate the benefits and burdens of AN&H to ensure quality of life is maintained (6,14, 23). Refer to Chapter 11, *Enteral Nutrition in Adult Medical/Surgical Oncology,* and Chapter 12, *Parenteral Nutrition in Medical/Surgical Oncology,* for specifics relating to enteral and parenteral nutrition, respectively.

Summary

Effective palliative nutrition therapy focuses on a patient's quality of life by using an interdisciplinary team approach to manage nutrition-related symptoms and to optimize nutrition status. Individual needs and wishes must be carefully determined when offering food and fluids to ensure the best possible comfort and enjoyment in the final stage of a person's life. The nutrition care plan needs to address the patient's medical status, informed preference, and the involved institution's policies on AN&H. The qualifications of the dietetics professional make him/her an essential part of the decision-making, education, and implementation process for any patient receiving AN&H.

References

1. American Cancer Society. Available at www.cancer.org. Accessed February 7, 2000.
2. Doyle D, Hanks G, Macdonald N. *Oxford Textbook of Palliative Medicine*. New York, NY: Oxford University Press; 1996.
3. Clothier J. Death and Dying. Syllabus for University of Arkansas for Medical Sciences. UAMS Dept of Psychiatry. Available at: http://www.uams.edu. Accessed August 15, 1998.
4. Gallagher-Allred C, O'Rawe Amenta M. *Nutrition and Hydration in Hospice Care; Needs, Strategies, Ethics*. New York, NY: The Haworth Press; 1993.
5. Levy MH, Rosen SM, Ottery FD, Hermann J. Supportive care in oncology. *Curr Probl Cancer*. 1992;16(6):329-418.
6. Gallagher-Allred C. *Nutritional Care of the Terminally Ill*. Rockville, Md: Aspen Publishers, Inc; 1989.
7. Donnelly S, Walsh D, Rybicki L. The symptoms of advanced cancer: identification of clinical and research priorities by assessment of prevalence and severity. *J of Pall Care*. 1995;11:27-32.
8. Kaye P. *Symptom Control In Hospice & Palliative Care*. 1st ed. Essex, Conn: Hospice Ed. Institute; 1994.
9. Shils M, Olson J, Shike M, Ross AC. *Modern Nutrition in Health and Disease*. 9th ed. Baltimore, Md: Williams and Willkins; 1999;1297-1325
10. Machlin L. *Handbook of Vitamins*. 2nd ed. New York, NY: Marcel Dekker Inc; 1991.
11. Walker MS, Masino K. *Oncology Nutrition Patient Education Materials*. Chicago, Ill: American Dietetic Association, 1998.
12. Madioni F, Morales C, Michel JP. Body image and the impact of terminal disease. *Eur J Pall Care*. 1997;4 (5):2-5.
13. Stevens EM. Promoting self-worth in the terminally ill. *Eur J Pall Care*. 1996;3(2):1-12
14. Burge F, Byock I, Daniels D, Mueller F, Schmale J, Williams C. Artificial Hydration and Nutrition in the terminally ill: a review. *Acad Hospice Physicians*. July 1995.
15. Burge F. Dehydration symptoms of palliative care cancer patients. *J Pain Symptom Manage* 1993;8(7):454-64.
16. Printz LA. Terminal dehydration, a compassionate treatment. *Arch of Int Med*. 1992;152:697-700.
17. Sullivan RJ. Accepting death without artificial nutrition or hydration. *J Gen Med*. 1993;8220-224.
18. McCamish M, Crocker N. Enteral and parenteral nutrition support of terminally ill patients: practical and ethical perspectives. *The Hospice Journal*. 1993;9(2/3):107-129.
19. Hospice Alliance Inc. *Palliative Care Guidelines*. Upstate New York, NY: 1997.
20. Gostin LO. Deciding life and death in the courtroom. From Quinlan to Cruzan, Glucksberg, and Vacco-a brief history and analysis of constitutional protection of the "right to die". *J Am Med Assoc*. Nov 12 1997;278(18):1523-1528.
21. Mosely K. Medical Ethics: Sometimes Less is More. "The art and science of managing patients requiring enteral and parenteral nutrition." 11th Annual Nutrition Symposium. Detroit, MI: U of D Mercy; Nov 1997.
22. Advance directives. American Health Care Association. Available at www.ahca.org. Accessed August 7, 1998.
23. Position of the American Dietetic Association. Issues in feeding the terminally ill adult. *J Am Diet Assoc*. 1992;92:996-1002.
24. Position of the American Dietetic Association: Issues in feeding permanently unconscious patients. *J Am Diet Assoc*. 1995;95:231-234.

16

Alternative Therapies in Oncology

Laura Molseed, MS, RD

The use of alternative therapies is becoming an increasingly popular and accepted practice among people with cancer (1). Alternative therapies are defined by the American Cancer Society (ACS) as "diagnostic tests or therapeutic modalities which are promoted for general use in cancer prevention, diagnosis, or treatment and which are, on the basis of careful review by scientists and/or other clinicians, not deemed proven nor recommended for current use" (2). "Alternative" implies that the therapy is utilized in place of conventional medicine. Today, many of these therapies are also known as "complementary" medicine, which implies that these treatments are used in addition to conventional treatment (3). This chapter focuses on the history of various therapies, their current use in cancer treatment, claims made about them, and the potential benefits and/or harms of each therapy.

Prevalence of the Use of Alternative Therapies

Eisenberg et al. estimated in 1993 that over $13 billion is spent annually on alternative medical treatments in the United States. Approximately one quarter of the persons with cancer polled reported using an alternative therapy before, during, or after their conventional oncologic treatment. Some of the most common treatments reported included various diet therapies, megavitamin supplementation, and herbal treatments (4). The individuals reporting the highest use were middle-aged, well-educated adults (4). The treatments varied greatly, as did the use and setting (see Box 16.1).

Box 16.1   Most Common Alternative Treatments

• Relaxation	• Lifestyle diets
• Chiropractic	• Herbal medicine
• Massage	• Megavitamin therapy
• Imagery	• Self-help groups
• Spiritual healing	• Energy healing
• Commercial weight loss programs	• Biofeedback
• Hypnosis	• Homeopathy
• Acupuncture	• Folk remedies

Rationale for Turning to Alternative Therapies

Although conventional cancer treatment has made significant progress in the treatment of cancer, cures are not guaranteed and the side effects of the treatment are often viewed as causing more harm than good. Many alternative therapies are marketed as non-toxic, safe, and "natural." People often believe that their cancer could have been prevented and is now curable by following a particular diet and lifestyle (3).

These treatments give people a sense of hope and allow them to feel as if they have an active role in their treatment (3).

Health professionals must develop a sound understanding of the various alternatives that are being utilized. Awareness of the potential health concerns surrounding each therapy as well as an understanding of the reasoning behind an individual's decision to use these treatments is essential for all health professionals. Health professionals should maintain open communication with patients and discuss the treatments they are investigating and any concerns about their conventional treatment.

Diet Therapies

Diet therapies, as a form of disease treatment, are some of the oldest and most commonly employed alternative treatments. Many people understand the role diet and various nutrients may have in cancer prevention, and may also feel that these same principles have a potential role in curing or reversing the carcinogenic process (1,3). Nutrition alone, however, has never been proven to cure or reverse a malignant process.

Vegetarianism

A vegan diet, and variations of it, are often employed as part of a metabolic program to help clear the body of toxins, or may be utilized alone as an adjunct to conventional cancer treatment. "Natural" and "organic" foods are often encouraged, and all animal products are eliminated (5). Often specific cooking methods and food preparation techniques are encouraged (5).

A vegetarian diet can be a healthful, nutrient-complete diet when coupled with proper education and careful meal planning. Individuals who have no difficulty eating or who are not experiencing treatment-related side effects may find these diets very acceptable. However, those individuals who are experiencing difficulty eating may not be able to obtain adequate nutrition. The use of alternate protein sources, medical nutritionals, and vitamin and mineral supplements should be encouraged with patients undergoing active cancer treatment. See Box 16.2 for nutrition and health concerns.

Box 16.2   Nutrition and Health Concerns with Vegetarian Diets

> - Protein deficiency
> - Vitamin B_{12} deficiency
> - Calcium, magnesium, zinc, and iron deficiency
>
> **Efficacy**
> - Diet is low in total fat and saturated fat.
> - Diet is rich in whole grains and fruit and vegetable fiber.
> - There is no scientific evidence to support the use of diet alone as a cancer treatment and currently no evidence to indicate that a vegetarian diet has a curative effect (1,5,6).

Macrobiotic Diet

The Kushi Institute and East West Foundation promote the macrobiotic diet and way of life as a treatment for all types of cancer. Their theory is that the majority of physical ailments experienced today are a result of poor nutrition and an unhealthy, unnatural lifestyle. They believe that the development of cancer is due to an overconsumption of excess yin or yang foods and to the body's constant attempt to rid itself of waste products (7).

Individuals who follow the macrobiotic principles believe in obtaining a balance with the food they eat and the environment in which they live (7, 8). The standard macrobiotic diet (Box 16.3) is similar to a strict vegetarian diet; all meats and dairy products are excluded and replaced with many soy-based products. Other items normally included in a vegetarian diet, such as citrus fruits and some vegetables, however, are often limited or excluded. Supplemental foods such as white meat fish, seasonal fruit, nuts, and seeds may be included two to three times a week. Vitamin and mineral supplementation is discouraged. Specialized cooking techniques and lifestyle changes are encouraged. In addition, special teas are the only beverage allowed, and are to be consumed only when thirsty. Depending on the type of cancer, the part of the body affected, and the climate in which the individual lives, the diet may vary and other foods may be limited or allowed in greater quantities. See Box 16.2 for nutrition and health concerns.

Box 16.3   Standard Macrobiotic Diet

Ranges
50% to 60% Whole grains
25% to 30% Vegetables
5% to 10% Soups
5% to 10% Beans and sea vegetables

Nutrition and Health Concerns with Macrobiotic Diet
- Protein deficiency
- Vitamin B_{12} deficiency
- Calcium deficiency
- Potential for dehydration
- Strong emotional burden placed on the individual and family

Efficacy
- The diet currently is being investigated for its potential cancer preventative effects.
- Soy products contain genistein, a potential cancer preventative agent.
- Antioxidants are under investigation for preventative effects as well as therapeutic effects.
- Many of the lifestyle changes are consistent with overall disease preventative recommendations
- There is no scientific evidence indicating this diet, used alone or as an adjunct to conventional therapy, cures cancer. (1,9)

Metabolic Therapy

Metabolic therapies are promoted on the assumption that cancer and other disease processes result from the buildup of toxins and waste products in the body. When the immune system, respiratory system, liver, and pancreas can no longer rid the body of these toxins, the body's normal metabolic processes are interrupted and chronic disease may occur (5). There are numerous variations and components of metabolic therapy regimes (Table 16.1), however, they all tend to follow the traditional three-step process of detoxification, fasting, and rejuvenation. They use "natural" and "organic" foods, vitamins, minerals, hormones, enzymes, enemas, laetrile, and various other treatments in their detoxification and rejuvenating process (5,10). Numerous variations of these treatments are normally offered in clinics in Mexico and the Bahamas. However, many aspects of the treatments may be done in the individual's home.

Dr. Max Gerson developed the original metabolic therapy, which claimed that following a system of purging and a strict nutrition program would cure cancer and other chronic diseases. His regimen, which is still offered in Mexico, encourages five coffee enemas a day to cleanse the body. It calls for 13 eight-ounce servings of fresh juice, three servings of calf liver juice, a bowl of oatmeal, a baked potato, raw

Table 16.1   Common Agents Utilized in Metabolic Programs

Therapy	Claim	Efficacy	Nutritional and Health Concerns
Coffee enemas	Detoxify the body. Enhance bile flow and excretion. (Rid the body of waste products) (5,10)	Does not detoxify the body. Does not enhance bile flow excretion. (9,11)	Fat and fat soluble vitamin malabsorption Electrolyte imbalances Dehydration Colonic perforation Infection (9,11)
Laetrile	Anticancer agent	Clinical trials at NCI found no benefit. (9)	Acute cyanide toxicity (especially when taken with Vitamin C or Vitamin C–containing foods) (9)
Pancreatic enzymes	Break down cancerous tissue	Only effective in people with malabsorption due to pancreatic insufficiency. Do not break down cancerous tissue.	Tissue breakdown around gastro-intestinal malignancies causing bleeding and gastrointestinal tract lining destruction. (5)
Glandular products	Help the affected organ function more effectively (5)	Glandular products are digested by the body, like protein. (5)	Contaminated samples have been reported. (5)

vegetables and fruit, and 2 tablespoons of linseed oil daily. Thyroid, a solution of iodine/potassium iodide, acidophilus, royal jelly, niacin, and a vitamin B_{12} injection are also prescribed. Other treatments including laetrile and rectal ozone may also be utilized depending on the disease. There have been numerous reports to various medical organizations of infection and deaths from this treatment and no demonstrated efficacy (11).

Another treatment, Cancell or Entelev, was introduced by James Sheridan and Edward Sopecak in the 1930s. It appears to be a nonstandardized chemical formulation that may consist of inositol, nitric acid, sodium sulfite, potassium hydroxide, sulfuric acid, and catechol. The promoters claim that this product will change the vibrational frequency and energy of the cancer cells, causing them to self-destruct and to be discharged from the body. In addition to internal and external treatments with the product, 1000 mg of bromelain before meals is prescribed, and a natural, preservative-free, vegetarian diet must be adhered to at all times. All other forms of cancer treatment are to be abandoned. Studies completed in the 1970s and 1980s at the National Cancer Institute on animals found this product to be ineffective in the treatment of cancer. The Food and Drug Administration has prohibited the manufacture and distribution of Cancell or Entelev in the United States (12).

Nutrient and Herbal Supplementation

The lure of "natural," "non-toxic," or "organic" treatment programs often leads consumers to herbal medicine and nutrient supplementation (1,13). Consumers rarely think of these products as potentially harmful because they are purchased over the counter and normally self-selected rather than prescribed by a physician (13,14). Nutrient and herbal supplements are regulated by the Dietary Supplement and Health and Education Act (DSHEA) of 1994. This act states:
• Products may be marketed without any efficacy testing.
• Products may be manufactured without following any standards.
• Claims are allowed on the package and product brochures as long as they are truthful and not misleading.
• Manufacturers do not need to prove that dietary supplements are safe. The Food and Drug Administration (FDA) is responsible for proving that they are unsafe before they can be taken off the market. (14)

Unfortunately, consumers do not understand these guidelines and often believe that any product sold as a pill or food has FDA backing and is safe for consumption (13).

Nutrient Supplementation

The most active and most commonly "self-prescribed" area of alternative medicine is nutrient supplementation. Megavitamin therapy alone or in combination with other treatments has become common practice among individuals with cancer. The media, including television, radio, newspapers, and the Internet, often publicize the effectiveness of various nutrients in the prevention and treatment of chronic disease, which confuses the public and adds to the questions asked of many health care providers (1). According to recent estimates, 50% of all Americans take some kind of nutrient supplement (15). Promoters of megavitamin therapy function under the belief that "if some is good, more is better," forgetting to or failing to warn the public about the potential harmful side effects of large doses of these nutrients. In addition, little research regarding the use of supplements has been done to evaluate how they may affect health (15). Table 16.2 reviews commonly recommended supplements, their efficacy, and nutrition and health-related concerns.

Table 16.2   Commonly Recommended Nutrient Supplements (16,17,18,19)

Vitamin	Efficacy	Nutritionist and Health-Related Concerns
Vitamin A RDA—800 g RE (adults)	Some forms of Vitamin A are undergoing investigation as an anticancer agent. There is no efficacy for dietary supplementation as a cancer treatment.	Intakes between 50,000 IU and 100,000 IU can cause nausea, vomiting, diminished appetite, weight loss, joint pain, abdominal discomfort, irritability, bone deformities, and hepatomegaly.
Beta Carotene No RDA established	May inhibit the growth of abnormal cells, strengthen immune response, fortify cell membranes, and alter abnormal cell production.	There are no known toxicities. Recent clinical trials revealed populations at high risk of developing lung cancer who received beta carotene supplementation had higher cancer rates.
Vitamin C RDA: 60 mg/day (adults)	Studies have shown no efficacy in the treatment of cancer.	Megadoses (2 g to 10 g a day) may cause diarrhea, dental erosion, clotting abnormalities, kidney stones, and low copper and selenium levels.
Vitamin E RDA: 8 mg alpha TE/day	There is currently no evidence to support megadoses as a cancer treatment. Vitamin E is an antioxidant and may have a role in cancer prevention.	Megadoses have the potential to interfere with the absorption of Vitamin K. Little other toxicity has been noted.
Selenium RDA: 55–70 mcg/day (adults)	Protects cell membranes from free radical damage. Effects seem to be enhanced with Vitamin E. Currently there is no evidence to support its use as a treatment for cancer.	Upper safe limit is 500 mcg/day. Prolonged intakes above 750 g/day may cause slowed growth, eye damage, hair loss, tooth decay, and compromised bone function.
Zinc RDA: 12–15 mg/day	Assists in immune enhancement and wound healing. May improve taste perception during radiation therapy. There is no evidence to suggest that megadoses will be of benefit in cancer treatment.	Intakes greater than 150 mg/day may suppress immune function. Intakes greater than 25 mg/day may impede copper absorption. High doses may cause nausea and vomiting.
Coenzyme Q10 (Ubiquinone)	Proponents claim that cancer patients lack CoQ10 in their blood and that it has a profound effect on the human immune system. There is no clinical evidence to support this and some studies indicate that it may enhance breast cancer cell growth.	There have been no toxic effects reported from CoQ10.

Another product that is marketed as a "nutritional supplement" and cancer treatment is shark cartilage. Biochemist William Lane, PhD has proposed that shark cartilage effectively inhibits angiogenesis, the formation of blood vessels, and thus inhibits the blood supply to tumors, limiting their ability to grow or metastasize. Numerous research studies are underway according to Lane and all are indicating positive responses (20). None of the studies reported to date, however, have undergone peer review; they have only been reported in the news media (21). Scientists are trying to isolate the protein in shark cartilage that may be responsible for inhibiting angiogenesis so they may investigate its antitumor properties. Controlled studies are needed before any claims can be made regarding the effectiveness of shark cartilage and they are currently underway (21).

Herbal Supplementation

Herbal treatments are most commonly sold as powders, pills, or teas. There are no Standards of Identity for herbal preparations and often the medicinal quality claimed is a very dilute form of the purified therapeutic agent. Herbal potency will vary depending upon the plant, species, growing and storage conditions, what part of the plant is used, and the preparation method employed (13). Preparations sold as powders or tablets often have so many other ingredients added to them in the processing that the resultant product may have little to none of the claimed medicinal constituent. In addition, preparations may contain other potentially harmful contaminants (13,22). Many companies are now claiming to manufacture their products according to their own established standards. The potential medicinal quality will still vary depending upon the plant species used, and conditions in which it is grown. There currently is no good way for consumers to know exactly what they are purchasing.

A number of herbal treatments have been utilized and marketed for the treatment of cancer and for symptom relief. It is important for health care professionals to understand the regulations surrounding these treatments, as well as the potential benefits and harms that may be caused by these products in order to guide and counsel their clients (13,22,23). Table 16.3 reviews some of the herbal products that cancer patients may hear about and try, the claims that have been made, and the safety and efficacy of the products, along with current recommendations.

Working with Patients

More people with cancer and their families are seeking information about available treatments for cancer. There is a wealth of information, both good and misleading, available through bookstores, health food stores, libraries, support groups, neighbors, friends, and the Internet. It is vitally important for health care professionals to have a working knowledge about alternative therapies and to be able to rationally discuss them with their patients (1,2,5,23,24).

Establish a good rapport with your patients. Talk openly and honestly about the therapies they have investigated. Listen to their reasoning and understand their need to have an active role in their treatment. Maintain a caring and sensitive attitude. It is important that they know that you are concerned about the effect their nutrition status has on their overall health, not just because of their cancer diagnosis (1,5,24).

Educate patients about the safety and health concerns related to the treatments they are investigating and how they can evaluate various claims for themselves. If a treatment won't hurt them, even if it has not been proven to be beneficial, it may be worth trying. If there are potential health concerns with a particular product or therapy, you need to let them know those concerns so they will be able to make educated decisions (1,5,24,25).

Make regular visits to health food stores and be knowledgeable about treatments that patients are investigating. Ask your patients where they received their information and if you could have a copy of it. Keep a library of books about alternative therapies for quick reference. (See Appendixes A and B.) Keep both legitimate and questionable publications handy. Your patients will appreciate your effort to learn about the therapies and will know that you are informing them of real concerns (1,5,25).

Respect your patients' hopes and desires to be an active part of their treatment. Encourage them to read and research treatments and to become knowledgeable about nutrition. Have them bring articles, books, and newsletters to you for review. Then point out both the potential beneficial aspects of the treatments and any potential harmful effects (1,5,25).

Table 16.3   Commonly Recommended Herbal Products (13,22,23)

Herb	Claim	Efficacy	Safety	Current Recommendations
Chaparrel	Analgesic Expectorant Diuretic Emetic Anti-inflammatory	Studies have shown no anticancer effect.	Long-term use in rats led to lesions in mesentary, lymph nodes, and kidneys. One documented case of liver disease in humans. Removed from the Generally Recommended as Safe (GRAS) list.	Not recommended.
Echinacea	Immune stimulant Wound healer	Widely used in Germany to treat the common cold and respiratory and urinary tract infections. Needs more research.	Significant side effects have not been observed. Allergies are always possible.	May be used with caution. Not recommended for longer than 8 consecutive weeks. Not recommended during pregnancy or lactation.
Essiac	Developed by Canadian nurse Rene Cassie to treat cancer	No anticancer effects.	Not safe for consumption and is illegal to distribute in the United States.	Not recommended.
Ginger	Digestive aid Stimulant Diuretic Antiemetic	Found to be useful in treating motion sickness. Antiemetic properties are due to the local action on the stomach, not on the central nervous system.	No toxicities have been reported. Very large overdoses may cause central nervous system depression and cardiac arrhythmias. Thrombocytopenia has been reported in people taking large doses.	May be used for temporary relief of nausea.
Hoxey herbs	Anticancer agent	No benefit has ever been documented. Note that the originator Harry Hoxey died of prostate cancer while treating himself with his formula.	Not recommended.	Not recommended.
Kombucha Tea (Manchurian Tea or Kargasok Tea)	Immune system stimulator	Unsubstantiated claims of antitumor activity.	Home-brewed "mushroom" usually passed to friends and family members. Susceptible to microbial contamination. Acidosis, aspergillosis, nausea, vomiting, and jaundice have been reported.	Not recommended.
Milkthistle	Liver protector (active ingredient is silymarin)	Appears to protect undamaged liver cells from toxins. May be helpful in cirrhosis and hepatitis.	No adverse effects have been noted.	Safe for use. May have beneficial effects.
Mistletoe (American and European)	American—stimulates smooth muscle, increases blood pressure, increases uterine and intestinal contractions European—decreases blood pressure, antispasmodic, calmative agent	Extracts of the European form have been used as a palliative cancer treatment. There is little evidence supporting effectiveness	Berries are poisonous, and some evidence suggests the leaves may also be poisonous.	Not recommended.
Pau d'arco	Powerful tonic Blood builder Anticancer agent Also used to treat diabetes, rheumatism, and ulcers	Has been shown to have activity against cancer in animals but causes severe side effects in humans.	Toxic—induces nausea, vomiting, anemia, and bleeding in humans.	Not recommended.
Peppermint	Digestive aid Antispasmodic	Stimulates bile flow Stimulates tonus of the lower esophageal sphincter Appetite stimulant	Safe for adults. Not recommended for children due to increased choking reflex with menthol.	Safe for adults. Not recommended for children.
Pokeroot	Cathartic Emetic Narcotic Anticancer Dyspepsia Glandular swelling	No efficacy has been demonstrated for any claim except that it is a strong emetic and cathartic.	Extremely toxic. Causes gastroenteritis, hypotension, and respiration. Fatal in children.	Not recommended.

Summary

Alternative therapies have been utilized for centuries, but their use today seems to be dramatically increasing. While research continues to offer glimmers of hope for a cancer cure in the future and more people are able to live long and productive lives with a cancer diagnosis, cancer still remains a devastating disease. It is easy to understand why many patients, as well as well-meaning family and friends, turn to anything that may provide comfort, a sense of control, and a feeling of hope.

Information about various treatments, including alternative therapies, is more accessible today than ever. Technology has put much of this information at our fingertips. In addition, individuals are taking a more proactive approach in making decisions about their medical care. Medical practitioners must be cognizant of this, must be aware of the treatments that their patients may be utilizing, and be willing to ask questions about those treatments. Taking time to listen and providing appropriate guidance regarding various treatment options, including those an individual may be seeking on their own, is a significant part of a practitioner's role in cancer care.

References

1. Cassileth BR, Chapman CC. Alternative and Complementary Cancer Therapies. *Cancer.* 1996;77(6):1026-1034.
2. McGinnis LS. Alternative Therapies, 1990. *Cancer.* 1991;67(suppl 6):1788-1792.
3. Schimpff SC. Complementary Medicine. *Curr Opin Onc.* 1997;9:327-331.
4. Eisenberg DM, Kessler RC, Foster C, Norlock FE, Calkins DR, Delbance TL. Unconventional Medicine in the United States. *N Engl J Med.* 1993;328:246-252.
5. Keeler A. Nutrition quackery and cancer treatment. *ON-LINE.* 1995;3(3):3-11.
6. The American Dietetic Association. Position of the American Dietetic Association: Vegetarian diets—technical support paper. *JADA.* 1988;88(3): 352-355.
7. Kushi M. *The Macrobiotic Approach to Cancer: Toward Preventing and controlling Cancer with Diet and Lifestyle.* 3rd ed. Garden City Park, Ny: Avery Publishing Group, Inc; 1991.
8. Miller DR, Specker BL, Ho ML Norman EJ. Vitamin B-12 status in a macrobiotic community. *Am J Clin Nutr.* 1991;53:524-529.
9. Guzley GJ. Alternative cancer treatments: Impact of unorthodox therapy on the patient with cancer. *South Med J.* 1992; 85(5):519-523.
10. Green S. A critique of the rational for cancer treatment with coffee enemas and diet. *JAMA.* 1992;268(22):3224-3227.
11. Unproven methods of cancer management: Gerson Method. Review. *CA Canc J Clin.* 1990;40(4):252-256.
12. Questionable methods of cancer management: Cancell/Entelev. Review. *CA Canc J Clin.* 1993;43(1):57-62.
13. Foster S and Tyler VE. *The Honest Herbal: A Sensible Guide to the Use of Herbs and Related Remedies.* 4th ed. Binghamton, Ny: The Haworth Press, Inc; 1998.
14. FDA published final dietary supplement rules. USDHHS Center for Food Safety and Applied Nutrition. FDA Talk Paper. Available at http://vm.cfsan.fda.gov/lrd/tpsupp2.html. Accessed September 23, 1997.
15. Patterson RE, White E, Kristal AR, Neuhouser ML Potter JD. Vitamin supplements and cancer risk: the epidemiologic evidence. *Cancer Causes and Control.* 1997;8:786-802.
16. Somer E. *The Essential Guide to Vitamins and Minerals.* New York, NY: Harper-Collins Publishers; 1995.
17. Kubena KS, McMurray DN. Nutrition and the immune system: a review of nutrient-nutrient interactions. *JADA.* 1996;96(11):1156-1164.
18. Larsson O. Effects of isoprenoids on growth of normal human mammary epithelial cells and breast cancer cells in vitro. *Anticancer Research.* 1994;14:123-128.
19. Lockwood K, Mordhsstf D, Folkers K. Partial and complete regression of breast cancer in patients in relation to dosage of coenzyme Q_{10}. *Biochemical and Biophysical Research Communications.* 1993;3:1504-1508.

20. Lane IW. Shark Cartilage: It's medical potential. *Health Freedom News*. 1992;72–74.
21. Hunt TJ, Connelly JF. Shark Cartilage for cancer treatment. *Am J Health Syst Pharm*. 1995;52:1756–1760.
22. Youngkin EQ, Israel DS. A review and critique of common herbal alternative therapies. *Nurse Pract*. 1996;21(10):39–62.
23. Spaudling-Albright N. A review of some herbal and related products commonly used in cancer patients. *ON-LINE*. 1997; 5(2):1–9.
24. Woodward, MA. Alternative Medicine: fraud or miracle cures? *Life in Med*. April 1993;16–21.
25. Eisenberg, DM Advising patients who seek alternative medical therapies. *Am Coll Phy*. 1997;127:61–69.

Resources for the Dietetics Professional

Books

Barrett S, Cassileth BR. (ed) The American Cancer Society. *Dubious Cancer Treatment: A Report on Alternative Methods and the Practitioners and Patients Who Use Them*. The American Cancer Society, Florida Division; 1991

Bisset NG, ed. *Herbal Drugs and Phytopharmaceuticals*. Boca Raton, Fl: CRC Press; 1994.

Blumenthal M, Goldberg A, Gruenwald J, Hall T, et al (eds). [Klein S, Rister RS (trans)]. *The Complete Commission E Monographs: Therapeutic Guide to Herbal Medicines*. (English Translation). Austin, Tex: American Botanical Council and Boston, Mass: Integrative Medicine Communications; 1998.

Robbers JE, Tyler VE. *Herbs of Choice*. 2nd ed. Binghamton, NY: The Haworth Press, Inc; 1998.

Foster S, Tyler VE. *The Honest Herbal*. 4th ed. Binghamton, NY: The Haworth Press, Inc; 1998.

Zwicky JF, Hafner AW, Barrett S, Jarvis WT. *Reader's Guide to Alternative Health Methods*. Milwaukee, WI: The American Medical Association; 1993.

Agencies

The American Cancer Society	1-800-ACS-2345	www.acs.com
The National Cancer Institute	1-800-4-CANCER (1-800-422-6237)	www.nci.nih.gov
The National Council Against Health Fraud	215-437-1795	www.ncahf.org
The American Dietetic Association	1-800-877-1600	www.eatright.org
The American Medical Association	1-800-464-5000	www.ama-assn.org
The Food and Drug Administration	1-800-FDA-4010 (1-800-332-4010)	www.fda.gov
The American Botanical Council	1-800-373-7105	www.herbalgram.org
The Herb Research Foundation	1-303-449-2265	www.herbs.org
NAPALERT (National Products Alert Database Program for Collaborative Research/Pharmaceutical Sciences College of Pharmacy)	1-312-996-2246	
The National Center for Complementary and Alternative Medicine Clearinghouse	1-888-644-6226	
NIH Office of Dietary Supplements	1-301-435-2920	http://odp.od.nigh.gov

Rosenthal Center for Alternative/   1-212-543-9550   www.cpmcnet.columbia.edu/
Complementary Medicine,   dept/rosenthal
Columbia University

Books Your Patients May Be Reading

Frahm A, Frahm D. *A Cancer Battle Plan: Six Strategies for Beating Cancer from a Recovered Hopeless Case*. Colorado Springs, Co: Pinon Press; 1992.

Kushi M. *The Macrobiotic Approach to Cancer: Toward Preventing and Controlling Cancer with Diet and Lifestyle*. Garden City Park, NY: Avery Publishing Group; 1991.

Patrick Quinlin, PhD, RD. *Beating Cancer with Nutrition*. Tulsa, Okla: Nutrition Times Press, Inc; 1994.

Pelton RPh, PhD, Lee Overholser PhD. *Alternatives in Cancer Therapy: The Complete Guide to Non-Traditional Treatments*. New York, NY: Simon and Schuster; 1994.

A multitude of books is available to the lay public. The books listed here are a small sample of what is available in most bookstore self-help or medical sections.

17

Nutrition During Cancer Recovery

Daniel W. Nixon, MD

Every living cell, plant or animal, normal or abnormal, requires adequate nutrition to survive. Normal nutrition promotes normal cellular activity, whereas nutrition abnormalities lead to deranged cellular functions and to clinical disease.

Data increasingly link nutrition to each of the stages of cancer development (initiation, promotion, and progression) (1). Macronutrients, micronutrients, and a host of phytochemicals that are not nutrients in the traditional sense can have powerful effects at the cellular and subcellular level, both as causative and as preventive agents.

This chapter focuses on the patient recovering from cancer (ie, those who have been treated for cure). Nutrition in the patient with advanced cancer and treatment related symptoms are discussed in Chapter 6, *Chemotherapy and Nutrition Implications,* Chapter 7, *Nutrition Concerns with the Radiation Therapy Patient,* Chapter 8, *Nutrition Implications of Surgical Oncology,* and Chapter 15, *Medical Nutrition Therapy in Palliative Care.*

Background

Specific connections between diet and cancer come from epidemiology and from laboratory research. For example, breast cancer is less common in Japan, and Japanese breast-cancer patients have better survival rates than patients in the United States; this observation, attributed to the traditional Japanese diet, which is very low in total fat, strengthens the dietary fat breast-cancer hypothesis. In the laboratory, evidence accumulated over the last 50 years indicates that dietary fat and energy can profoundly affect the growth and development of carcinogen-induced tumors, including breast cancer, in animals (2,3,4). In a recent review, Torosian discussed parenteral and enteral nutrition experiments in animals and pointed out that such non-volitional feeding was associated with significant acceleration of tumor growth in breast cancer, sarcoma, hepatoma and other tumor models (5). Fewer data are available from human study, and information regarding tumor growth stimulation with nutritional support is inconclusive.

Human cancer cells implanted in animals and also grown in-culture can be profoundly influenced by exposure to certain nutrients and phytochemicals. Implanted human prostate cancer cells may be stimulated to grow by linoleic acid, whereas implanted human breast cancer cells in mice were suppressed by a diet high in omega-3 fatty acids (6,7,8). Certain human cancer cells in-culture undergo growth arrest and apoptosis when exposed to a phytochemical found in raspberries called ellagic acid (9).

The cancer cell is subject to a variety of nutritional influences, both positive and negative, so that a patient with cancer presents challenges different from patients who do not have cancer. Complex interactions occur between the tumor, the host, the various treatments given, and the foods eaten. The type of tumor and its extent are important variables, as are any anatomic alterations resulting from the primary (usually surgical) treatment. Finally, it must be remembered that every patient, regardless of tumor type, is different, with individual metabolic needs, body composition, and ability to assimilate nutrients.

Recommendations and Rationale

Several of the most common types of cancer have been linked to diet. These include both cancers of squamous cell origin as well as those arising from glandular tissues (adenocarcinomas). Lung cancer, the most common malignancy worldwide, even though clearly related to tobacco use, has dietary associations as well. The risk of squamous cancers, e.g., lung, esophagus, mouth, and pharynx, is decreased in populations consuming diets high in vegetables and fruits. The risk of various adenocarcinomas (breast, prostate, colorectal) is related in varying degree to diets high in total and saturated fat. Because diets high in vegetables and fruit are likely to be low in total fat (and vice versa), the actual contribution to cancer risk from individual food components remains elusive. *Food, Nutrition and the Prevention of Cancer: A Global Perspective* provides a very complete review and discussion of this entire area (1).

Based on the known natural history of cancer and the dietary relationships mentioned above, several assumptions can be made:

1. A cancer patient treated for cure may still harbor undetected primary or disseminated cancer cells.
2. A "cured" cancer patient is at increased risk for other primary cancers in the same organ or in other organs.
3. Dietary measures that are good for general health promotion and cancer prevention (decreased total fat, increased vegetables, fruits, and grains) are also appropriate for recovering cancer patients, as is weight control through exercise and decreased total calorie consumption.
4. Any dietary regimen should, therefore, be designed to: a) limit the possibility of stimulating the growth and spread of any remaining tumor cells; and b) provide maximum prevention against new primary tumors.

It is not logical to provide a nutrition plan for a recovering cancer patient that emphasizes foods and nutrients that may have been involved in promoting the primary tumor. Obesity, high fat diets, and low consumption of vegetables and fruits have all been implicated as cancer risk factors, but the optimal dietary levels for fat, fiber, and phytochemicals are not certain. Realizing that such data are incomplete, and that major uncertainties also exist as to the risk/benefit ratios of various fat categories (saturated, polyunsaturated, monounsaturated), the following guidelines are reasonable for most recovering cancer patients with intact gastrointestinal function. These recommendations cannot be achieved overnight. The patient will need encouragement and education about label reading, serving sizes, food preparation, and the overall rationale for a high-fiber, low-fat, abundant vegetable, fruit, and grain eating plan. Standard tables and formulas can be used to determine more specific individual fat and calorie consumption goals. Over time, patients will not need to count calories and fat grams as they become accustomed to the new eating plan. In the Cancer Risk Reduction Clinic at the Hollings Cancer Center in Charleston, South Carolina, periodic four-day diet diaries have been very useful tools for initial evaluation and follow-up. Recovering cancer patients are, in general, very motivated to follow nutrition advice. They should be encouraged to make dietary changes slowly so they will not feel deprived of any particular food or amount of food (10). Skilled dietetic professionals are crucial to a patient's success in this effort.

Recommendations

1. Limit total fat intake to 15% to 20% of total calories. Monounsaturated fats are preferred over polyunsaturated and saturated fats within this overall goal.
2. Aim for 10 to 12 daily servings* of whole vegetables and fruits. Assuming about two grams of fiber per serving, this will provide about 20 grams of daily fiber and many anticancer phytochemicals. Be sure to eat a variety of these foods.
3. Consume 4 to 6 servings* of whole grains daily. Alternatively, one serving of a high-fiber cereal is acceptable. This recommendation will add about 10 grams of fiber to the amount recommended in the preceding point, to reach a level of about 30 grams of fiber daily.
4. Breast cancer patients should consider eliminating or severely restricting alcohol intake (1 to 2 drinks/week or less). Alcohol is now recognized as a contributor to breast cancer risk.

5. Consider a vitamin E supplement of 200 IU/day. This will replace any deficit of vitamin E from a reduced fat intake.
6. A standard dose multivitamin/mineral supplement daily is acceptable, if desired (not to exceed 100% of USRDA). Discuss supplement use with a physician. Supplements cannot and should not replace foods that contain cancer-fighting substances.
7. Exercise moderately. A 30-minute daily walk at a comfortable pace is good, as are swimming, biking, or a number of other alternatives. A patient should talk with his or her physician before starting an exercise program.
8. Maintain a desirable body weight.
   * Consult standard references for serving sizes.

Rationale

The core of these recommendations is limitation of fat energy intake and increased consumption of fruits, vegetables, and grains. A high-calorie, high-fat diet provides excess energy that may, in the absence of sufficient exercise, be deposited as body fat. Adipose cells can convert adrenal androgens to estrogens that may stimulate hormonally sensitive cancer cells. Furthermore, laboratory evidence implicates certain dietary fatty acids as stimulators of breast and prostate cancer cells in vitro (6,7,8). In patients, weight gain during adjuvant breast cancer therapy is not uncommon (11). Increased body fat can lead to potentially harmful increases in circulating estrogens, as mentioned. A higher relapse rate has been noted in breast cancer patients who gain weight (12).

Prior to diagnosis, obesity is a recognized breast cancer risk factor (also for prostate, endometrial, and several other cancers). A recent study showed that weight gain after age 20 substantially increases post-menopausal breast cancer risk (13). After diagnosis of breast cancer, increased body weight is associated with a shorter disease-free interval and decreased overall survival (14,15). Evidence thus suggests that obesity increases breast cancer risk and worsens prognosis after diagnosis.

The recommended fat intake is 15% to 20% of total calories. Such an intake reduces caloric load, decreases potentially harmful fatty acid intake, and by promoting weight loss, may inhibit hormonally sensitive cancers such as breast cancer by reducing the level of circulating estrogenic hormones. This is the fat intake level being used in the Womens Intervention Nutrition Study (WINS) breast cancer recurrence prevention protocol which has currently accrued over 1400 women to either a 15% versus a 30% fat intake arm. Clinical trial experience in breast cancer patients indicates that sustained decreases in fat intake and increases in vegetable, fruit, and fiber intake can be achieved with dietary counseling (16,17).

Vegetables, fruits, and grains contain hundreds of potentially cancer-suppressive phytochemicals (18). One of these phytochemicals, ellagic acid, which is found in raspberries, strawberries, other fruits, and many plants, has definite growth-inhibiting and apoptosis-inducing properties in cultured human cervix cancer cells (9). Other phytochemicals have anti-oxidant, anti-angiogenic, anti-hormonal, and carcinogen-neutralizing properties (18). A diet high in fruits and vegetables, eaten regularly and in variety, provides all these potentially helpful substances to the recovering cancer patient. The fiber in such a diet can have additional anti-cancer activity by lowering intestinal carcinogen contents and by decreasing the time for digestive contents to traverse the gut, thereby limiting the contact of the gut mucosa to luminal toxins. These beneficial phytochemicals are best obtained from whole foods, not from supplements/pills.

Future Needs

Much more research is needed regarding the roles of specific foods, such as soy products, and of individual fruits and vegetables as cancer modulators. Well-characterized phytochemicals (ie, phytoestrogens, ellagitannins, polyphenols) may eventually be genetically engineered to higher levels in fruits and vegetables. Candidate phytochemicals for clinical trials include the isoflavone genistein which is found in soybeans and has weak anti-hormonal activity in animal models; other potentially useful compounds are alpha-tocopherol, selenium, calcium, and non-nutrients such as ellagic acid. The importance of clinical trial testing of chemopreventive agents was well demonstrated in the alpha-tocopherol, beta carotene cancer prevention study, which attempted to decrease lung cancer in 29,000 Finnish smokers (19). Two unexpected results occurred: prostate cancer was decreased with alpha-tocopherol, and lung cancer was actually increased in the beta carotene group. Further well-conducted clinical trials will be crucial to create disease-specific nutrition guidelines.

Summary

The relationship between nutrition and cancer prevention is well known. The patient recovering from cancer treatment should review his or her diet habits to see how closely they resemble those described in this chapter. Changes in a patient's eating plan will not occur overnight, and skilled dietetic professionals are crucial to success. More research is needed to determine the link between diet and cancer recovery.

References

1. World Cancer Research Fund/American Institute for Cancer Research Panel (Potter JD, chair). Diet and the cancer process. In: *Food, Nutrition and the Prevention of Cancer: A Global Perspective*. World Cancer Research Fund/American Institute for Cancer Research; 1997: 54–71.
2. Morrison AS, Lowe CR, Macmahon B. Incidence, risk factors and survival in breast cancer: report on 5 years of follow-up observation. *Eur J Cancer*. 1977;13:209–214.
3. Tannenbaum A. The genesis and growth of tumors, II: effects of a high fat diet. *Cancer Res*. 1942;2:468–475.
4. Birt DF, Kris ES, Choe M, Pelling JC. Dietary, energy and fat effects on tumor promotion. *Cancer Res*. 1992;52(Suppl):2035–2039.
5. Torosian MH. Feeding the tumor: fact or fiction. *Cancer Prev Int*. 1998;3(2):93–98.
6. Rose DP, Connolly JM. Effects of fatty acids and eicosanoid synthesis inhibitors on the growth of two human prostate cancer cell lines. *Prostate*. 1991;18:243–254.
7. Clinton SK, Palmer SS, Spriggs CE, et al. Growth of the Dunning transplantable prostate adenocarcinoma in rats fed diets with various fat contents. *J Nutri*. 1988;118:908–914.
8. Rose DP, Connolly JM. Effects of dietary omega-3 fatty acids on human breast cancer growth and metastases in nude mice. *J Natl Cancer Inst*. 1993;85:1743–1747.
9. Narayanan BA, Geoffroy O, Willingham MC, et al. p53/p21 expression and its possible role in GI arrest and apoptosis in ellagic and treated cancer cells. *Cancer Letters*. 1999;136:215–221.
10. Nixon DW. *The Cancer Recovery Eating Plan*. New York, NY: Random House, Times Books; 1996.
11. Foltz AT. Weight gain among stage II breast cancer patients: a study of five factors. *Oncol Nurse Forum*. 1985;12:21–26
12. Camoriano JK, Loprinzi CL, Ingle JN, et al. Weight change in women treated with adjuvant therapy or observed following mastectomy for node positive breast cancer. *J Clin Oncol*. 1990;8:1327–1334.
13. Huang Z, Hankinson SE, Colditz GA, et al. Dual effects of weight and weight gain on breast cancer risk. *JAMA*. 1997;278:1407–1411.
14. Donegan WL, Hartz DJ, Rimm AA. The association of body weight with recurrent carcinoma of the breast. *Cancer*. 1978;41:1590–1594.
15. Newman SC, Miller AB, Howe GR. A study of the effect of weight and dietary fat on breast cancer survival time. *Am J Epidemiol*. 1986;123:767–774.
16. Pierce JP, Faerber S, Wright FA, et al. Feasibility of a randomized trial of a high-vegetable diet to prevent breast cancer recurrence. *Nutr and Cancer*. 1997;28:282–288.
17. Kristal AR, Shattuck AL, Bowen DJ, et al. Feasibility of using volunteer research staff to deliver and evaluate a low-fat dietary intervention: the American Cancer Society Breast Cancer Dietary Intervention Project. *Cancer Epidemol Biomarkers & Prev*. 1997;6(6):459–67.
18. Nixon DW, ed. *Chemoprevention of Cancer*. Boca Raton, FL: RC Press; 1994.
19. The Alpha-Tocopherol, Beta Carotene Cancer Prevention Study Group. The effect of vitamin E and beta carotene on the incidence of lung cancer and other cancer in male smokers. *NEJM*. 1994;330:1029–1035.

Appendix A

Suggested Management of
Nutrition-Related Symptoms

Marnie Dobbin, MS, RD   **Virginia W. Hartmuller, PhD, MS, RD, FADA**

This table contains suggestions which the dietetics professional may offer to help manage common nutrition-related symptoms associated with cancer and cancer treatment. It is important to remember that each person is unique. Some individuals may experience mild, transient discomforts, while others may be markedly affected by a wide spectrum of symptoms. Before implementing dietary suggestions, it is important to assess the patient's nutritional status. The Scored PG-SGA (see Chapter 2) is an excellent tool for this purpose. The *Oncology Nutrition Patient Education Materials* offer further suggestions and single-page handouts (1).

Table App A   Suggested Management of Nutritional Symptoms Experienced by the Cancer Patient (2,3,4)

Symptom	Nutrition Problems	Suggestions for the Patient
Altered Taste	Decreased oral intake, often resulting in weight loss	Choose appealing foods; consider the smell, texture, and appearance.
		If red meat tastes strange, substitute poultry, fish, eggs, dairy products, beans, tofu, or soymilk.
		Add spices, bacon, or onion to enhance the flavor of foods.
		Eat foods at room temperature or chilled.
		Avoid any foods that have an unpleasant taste.
		Use plastic utensils instead of stainless flatware to avoid a metallic taste.
		Add a small amount of instant decaffeinated coffee powder when commercial liquid nutrition supplements taste too sweet. Try an unflavored enteral product with added flavoring agents to produce sour, bitter, salty, or mint taste.
		Sip gingerale, suck on hard candy, or add freshly squeezed lemon juice to offset a bad taste.
		Practice regular mouth care, including brushing and rinsing with a mixture of 1 tsp. baking soda and $\frac{1}{2}$ cup water.

continued

Symptom	Nutrition Problems	Suggestions for the Patient
Anorexia	Weight Loss, cachexia	Choose high protein, high calorie foods to get the most out of what you eat.
		Limit beverages at mealtime to prevent feeling too full. Drink liquids between meals instead, and try milkshakes or other liquid supplements throughout the day.
		Think of food as a medicine and try to eat at scheduled times instead of waiting until hunger sets in.
		Change time, place, and surroundings of meals; eat slowly.
		Keep healthful snacks handy.
		Try exercise after meals to help promote appetite.
		Ask a doctor whether appetite stimulants may be appropriate.
Constipation	Uncomfortable GI disturbance such as abdominal pain and distention; decreased appetite. Severe constipation can result in nausea or vomiting and diarrhea.	Drink plenty of liquids (ie, water, soup, prune and other juices, or popsicles) between meals. A minimum of $1/2$ oz/per lb body weight is suggested.
		Increase physical activity as tolerated.
		Take a hot drink about $1/2$ hour before the time a bowel movement usually occurs.
		Slowly, progressively, increase high-fiber foods, such as fruits, vegetables, and legumes.
		Progressively add wheat bran to the diet, along with adequate liquids. Begin using two heaping tablespoons of wheat bran a day for three days and increase by 1 Tb. a day for three days until constipation is relieved. Do not exceed 6 Tb. in one day. Ways to incorporate wheat bran to foods: add to hot and cold cereals, applesauce, pudding, pancake and muffin batters, or sprinkle over casseroles.
Diarrhea	Dehydration with loss of electrolytes and malabsorption of nutrients	Eliminate greasy, fatty, or fried foods.
		Avoid gassy or irritating high-fiber foods and foods containing strong spices.
		Consume small amounts of food and liquids throughout the day instead of limiting intake to mealtimes.
		Drink plenty of fluids. Try room-temperature, mild liquids, such as water. Avoid excessive amounts of sweet beverages, ie, juices, fruit drinks, sport drinks, or sodas.
		Limit foods containing caffeine, such as coffee and some cola beverages.
		Restrict milk and dairy products to see if symptoms are alleviated. If so, low-lactose products or lactase enzyme products may be tried.
		Increase foods containing potassium, such as potatoes, bananas, or melons if diarrhea is severe.
		When malabsorption due to fat or lactose, or another food intolerance has been diagnosed, use appropriate enzyme replacements such as pancreatic enzymes/lipase or lactase products.
Difficulty swallowing (dysphagia)	Decreased intake of foods	Try sucking on hard candy or popsicles.
		Use soft or pureed foods; add gravy or sauces to foods to ease swallowing.
		Use products, such as analgesics (as recommended by your physician) for temporary relief.

continued

Symptom	Nutrition Problems	Suggestions for the Patient
Dry mouth (xerostomia)	Difficulty chewing and swallowing food; decreased intake of foods	Try very sweet or tart foods and beverages, which may stimulate saliva.
		Take frequent sips of water and try sucking on ice chips.
		Use products that moisten lips or that coat the mouth (such as artificial saliva).
		Try fruit nectar instead of juice.
		Use a straw to drink liquids.
		Practice regular mouth care, including brushing and rinsing with a mixture of 1 tsp. baking soda and 1/2 cup water.
Mouth sores or mucositis	Decreased intake of foods; weight loss	Cook foods until they are soft and tender. Cut food into small pieces, or puree it in a blender.
		Mix foods with gravy or sauces to make them easier to swallow.
		Supplement meals with high-calorie, high-protein drinks.
		Use a straw to direct fluids away from painful areas of the mouth or use a syringe to squirt liquids into the throat (the guidance of a speech pathologist may help).
		Avoid alcohol, caffeine, tobacco, and chemical irritants, such as citric acid, tomatoes, or hot peppers.
		Try numbing the mouth with ice chips or popsicles.
		Use good dental practices; use appropriate non-alcohol-containing mouth rinses. Try rinsing with a mixture of 1 tsp. baking soda mixed with 1/2 cup water.
		Check with a physician to see if this discomfort can be relieved by medications.
Nausea and vomiting	Decreased oral intake that may result in weight loss	Use an antiemetic to control nausea. If an anti-nausea medicine does not work, let your healthcare professional know so a more effective one may be found.
		Avoid taking beverages with foods because that might distend the stomach. Wait more than 15 minutes after eating before drinking liquids.
		Avoid fatty or spicy foods or foods with strong odors; try plain, starchy foods like potatoes, hot cereal, crackers, and pretzels.
		Eat slowly and consume small amounts often; try crackers, dry toast, or gingerale.
		Drink or sip liquids throughout the day.
		Try ginger ale, ginger tea, or crystallized ginger to help the nausea.
		Eat foods at room temperature or cooler because the aromas of hot foods may add to nausea.
		Avoid lying down for about one hour after eating; lying down may increase nausea and reflux.
		Avoid eating one to two hours before treatment; avoid eating favorite foods when feeling nauseous to discourage an aversion.
		When vomiting is controlled, first try small amounts of liquids and then add plain starchy foods like noodles or saltine crackers which are easily digested.
		Try taking a short walk to help empty the stomach. Slow emptying of the stomach can contribute to nausea.

continued

Symptom	Nutrition Problems	Suggestions for the Patient
Weight gain	Associated with other health risks; psychologic impact of self-image of body	If weight gain exceeds 5% to 10% of usual weight, seek counseling to manage weight.
		Exercise is encouraged unless it is contraindicated.
		Eat a well-balanced diet and eat at least five servings a day of fruits and vegetables.
		Identify high-calorie foods and consider eliminating them or reducing portion sizes.
		Reduce fats used at the table and in food preparation.
		Avoid quick-weight-loss diets.
		Discuss with your healthcare professional the relationship of diet and weight to other health risks.
		Try to identify emotional and environmental reasons for overeating and snacking.
Weight loss	Cachexia; electrolyte abnormalities; impaired organ function ; immuno-suppression	Take liquids between meals and try milkshakes or other liquid supplements.
		Eat whenever hungry; try small, frequent meals; avoid filling up on low calorie foods.
		Keep healthy snacks readily available like dried fruit, yogurt, custard, pudding, or cottage cheese.
		Choose high-protein, high-calorie foods to get the most out of the foods you eat.
		Eat small amounts of food and liquids throughout the day instead of limiting intake to mealtime.
		Increase calories by adding fat and other calorie-dense foods to the diet; try ice cream, cheese, and canned fruit in heavy syrup.
		Add whole milk or dry milk solids to recipes.
		To increase calories without changing the taste of food, add a glucose polymer supplement to beverages, soup, or gravies.
		Add modular protein supplements to increase nutritional value without increasing the volume of food.

References

1. Walker MS, Masino K, *Oncology Nutrition Patient Education Materials*. Chicago, Ill: The American Dietetic Association;1998.
2. Shils ME, Nutrition and diet in cancer management. In: Shils M, Olson, Shike, eds. *Modern Nutrition in Health and Disease*. Philadelphia, PA: Lippincott;1994:1317-1347.
3. PDQ: the National Cancer Institute's computerized database. Bethesda, MD: National Cancer Institute; date unknown; cited 1998 Feb 9. Available from: http://cancernet.nci.nih.gov/clinpdq/supportive/Nutrition_Physician.html.
4. Ottery FD. Definition of standardized nutritional assessment and interventional pathways in oncology. *Nutrition*. 1996;12(suppl):15S-19S.

Appendix B

Common Supportive Drug Therapies Used with Oncology Patients

LeAnne D. Kennedy, PharmD

Appendix B presents information about the common supportive drug therapies used with oncology patients in two different formats:
- in a textual format that summarizes the mechanism of action, indication, side effects, and available preparations
- in following tables, for ease-of-use

Information is included on the following drug therapies:

Antiemetic Agents Phenothiazines, Butyrophenones, Substituted Benzamides, Serotonin Antagonists, Benzodiazepines, Corticosteroids, Anticholinergics, Cannabinoids

Anti-diarrheal Agents Bulk-forming Agents, Anti-motility Agents, Other Agents, Codeine Derivatives

Laxatives Stool Softeners, Stimulants, Bulk-forming Agents, Hyperosmotic Laxatives, Saline Laxatives

Agents for Oral Care Cleansing Agents, Healing/Coating Agents, Topical Anesthetics, Analgesic Agents, Mucositis Mouthwashes, Antifungal Agents

Pain Medications Non-opioid Analgesics, Non-steroidal Anti-inflammatory drugs (NSAIDs), Opioids

Miscellaneous Agents Saliva Stimulants, Appetite Stimulants, Pancreatic Enzymes

Antiemetic Agents

Oncology patients experience nausea and vomiting for a variety of reasons including chemotherapy, radiation, and disease involvement. Antiemetics offer these patients relief from their symptoms and are most effective when used to prophylactically rather than to treat existing nausea and/or vomiting. Combining two or more drugs from different classes has been found to be beneficial while minimizing side effects. The serotonin antagonists in combination with corticosteroids are effective in the prevention of acute nausea and vomiting with highly emetogenic chemotherapy. Most decisions concerning choice of antiemetic are based on the emetogenicity of the chemotherapy. Serotonin antagonists are usually reserved for high and moderately high emetogenic chemotherapy. Phenothiazine and metoclopramide are effective for mild to moderate emetogenic chemotherapy. See table App B1 for selected drugs and classes that are used as antiemetics.

Note: Over-the-counter preparations are indicated by asterisk (**).
Side effects that have nutritional implications are underlined.
When recommending administration of a medicine down a nasogastric or Dobhoff tube, please consult your pharmacist because many medications have special considerations.

Phenothiazines

Mechanism of Action: block dopamine receptors in the chemoreceptor trigger zone (CTZ)
Indication: used primarily as prophylaxis against mild to moderately emetogenic chemotherapy.
Side Effects: extrapyramidal symptoms (EPS), sedation, hypersensitivity, hypotension

Prochlorperazine (Compazine®)
capsule, sustained action: 10 mg, 15 mg, 30 mg
injection: 5 mg/ml
suppository: 2.5 mg, 5 mg, 25 mg
syrup: 5 mg/5 ml
tablet: 5 mg, 10 mg, 25 mg

Promethazine (Phenergan®)
injection: 25 mg/ml; 50 mg/ml
suppository: 12.5 mg, 25 mg, 50 mg
syrup: 6.25/5 ml
tablet: 12.5 mg, 25 mg, 50 mg

Perphenazine (Trilafon®)
concentrate: 16 mg/5 ml
injection: 5 mg/ml
tablet: 2 mg, 4 mg, 8 mg, 16 mg

Thiethylperazine (Torecan®)
injection: 5 mg/ml
suppository: 10 mg
tablet: 10 mg

Butyrophenones

Mechanism of Action: dopamine receptor antagonist
Indication: used most often with moderate to severely emetogenic chemotherapy
Side Effects: sedation, dystonic reactions

Haloperidol (Haldol®)
concentrate: 2 mg/ml
injection: 5 mg/ml
tablet: 0.5 mg, 1 mg, 2 mg, 5 mg, 10 mg, 20 mg

Droperidol (Inapsine®)
injection: 2.5 mg/ml

Substituted Benzamide

Mechanism of Action: blocks dopamine receptors in the CTZ and peripherally; peripherally, increases esophageal sphincter tone, improves gastric emptying, and increases transit through the small bowel due to release of acetylcholine
Indication: very effective in large doses (2 mg/kg), most likely due to inhibition of serotonin receptors in addition to dopamine receptors
Side Effects: EPS (3-31%), restlessness, drowsiness, fatigue, nausea, and diarrhea

Metoclopramide (Reglan®)
injection: 5 mg/ml
solution, concentrated: 10 mg/ml
syrup, sugar free: 5mg/5 ml
tablet: 5 mg, 10 mg

Serotonin Antagonists

Mechanism of Action: blocks serotonin receptors peripherally through the enterochromaffin cells in the upper gastrointestinal tract or in the area postrema located in the CTZ
Indication: used for acute nausea and vomiting with little effect on delayed <u>nausea</u> and vomiting
Side Effects: headache, <u>constipation</u>, <u>diarrhea</u>, somnolence, EKG changes

Dolasetron (Anzemet®)
tablet: 50 mg, 100 mg
injection: 100mg/5 ml

Ondansetron (Zofran®)
tablet: 4 mg, 8 mg
injection: 2 mg/ml

Granisetron (Kytril®)
tablet: 1 mg
injection: 1 mg/ml

Benzodiazepines

Mechanism of Action: may interfere with afferent nerves from the cerebral cortex
Indication: used more for anticipatory nausea and vomiting, anxiety
Side Effects: sedation, decreased respiration, confusion, amnesia, slurred speech

Lorazepam (Ativan®)
tablet: 0.5 mg, 1 mg, 2 mg
injection: 2 mg/ml, 4 mg/ml
solution, concentrated: 2 mg/ml

Valium (Diazepam®)
tablet: 2 mg, 5 mg, 10 mg
injection: 5 mg/ml
solution: 5 mg/ 5 ml

Corticosteroids

Mechanism of Action: unknown, may inhibit prostaglandin synthesis
Indication: most effective when combined with dopamine or serotonin antagonists
Side Effects: <u>increased appetite</u>, mood changes, anxiety, euphoria, headache, <u>metallic taste,</u> abdominal discomfort, <u>hyperglycemia</u>

Dexamethasone (Decadron®)
tablet: 0.25 mg, 0.5 mg, 1 mg, 1.5 mg, 2 mg,
    4 mg, 6 mg
elixir: 0.5 mg/5 ml
injection: 4 mg/ml, 10 mg/ml

Anticholinergics

Mechanism of Action: blocks acetylcholine at the emetic center
Indication: used most when nausea is refractory and related to motion
Side Effects: urinary retention, dry eyes, <u>constipation</u>

Scopolamine (Trans Derm®)
topical patch: 1.5 mg

Cannabinoids

Mechanism of Action: unknown
Indication: used to prevent nausea and vomiting; well tolerated in younger patients
Side Effects: mood changes, <u>increased appetite</u>, hypotension, tachycardia, blurred vision

Dronabinol (Marinol®)
capsule: 2.5 mg, 5 mg, 10 mg

Table App B1   Antiemetics

Class	Drug	Oral	Rectal	Injectible	Mechanism of Action	Site of Action	Side Effects	Comments
Phenothiazines	Perphenazine (Trilafon)	x		x	DA	CTZ	EPS, sedation, hypotension	Prochlorperazine is the most effective agent in this class; perphenazine may be effective with high IV doses; prochlorperazine is available in sustained released capsule which should not be crushed.
	Prochlorperazine (Compazine)	x	x	x				
	Promethazine (Phenergan)	x	x	x				
	Thiethylperazine (Torecan)	x	x	x				
Butyrophenones	Droperidol (Inapsine)	x		x	DA	CTZ	EPS, sedation	
	Haloperidol (Haldol)	x	x	x				
Substituted Benzamide	Metoclopramide (Reglan)	x	x	x	DA or 5HT$_3$ in high doses	CTZ	EPS, sedation, fatigue, diarrhea, nausea	Also used in early satiety and anorexia
Seratonin Antagonists	Dolasetron (Anzemet)	x		x	5HT$_3$	CTZ, PGSEC	Headache, diarrhea, constipation, EKG changes, somnolence	Increased effect with coricosteroid
	Granisetron (Kytril)	x		x			Headache, diarrhea, constipation, somnolence	
	Ondansetron (Zofran)	x		x				
Benzodiazepines	Lorazepam (Ativan)	x		x	BDZ	Unknown	Sedation, confusion, amnesia, slurred speech	Effective for anticipatory nausea/anxiety; lorazepam may be placed under the tongue
	Diazepam (Valium)	x		x				
Corticosteroids	Dexamethasone (Decadron)	x		x	Unknown	Unknown	Increased appetite, mood change, anxiety, euphoria, headache, metallic taste, hyperglycemia	Most effective when used with 5HT$_3$
Anticholinergics	Scopolamine (TransDerm)		Patch		ACH	Emetic Center	Urinary retention, dry eyes, constipation	Effective for nausea related to motion
Cannabinoids	Dronabinol (Marinol)	x			Unknown	CNS	Mood changes, increased appetite, hypotension, tachycardia	Well tolerated in younger patients; may crush

Key: 5HT$_3$ = Seratonin antagonist; CTZ = Chemoreceptor trigger zone; DA = Dopamine antagonist; EPS = Extrapyramidal Side Effects; PGSEC = Peripheral Gastrointestinal Stimulation to Emetic Center

Anti-diarrheals and Laxatives

Diarrhea and constipation may pose problems for oncology patients. These problems may be related to disease, treatment, or side effects from other related therapies. Some agents such as calcium polycarbophil (Fibercon®) may be used as both an anti-diarrheal and a laxative. Caution should be used when recommending anti-diarrheals because diarrhea may be related to an infection and antimotility agents may cause harm to the patient. See Table App B2 for selected drugs and classes used as anti-diarrheals or laxatives.

Anti-diarrheals

Bulk-forming Agents

Mechanism of Action: absorbs water from the intestine to promote peristalsis
Side Effects: <u>bowel obstruction</u>, <u>diarrhea</u>, <u>constipation</u>, <u>abdominal cramps</u>

*Psyllium (Metamucil®, Citrucel®)**
   granules, powder, chewable squares, wafers

*Attapulgite (Kaopectate®)**
   chewable tablets, liquid

*Calcium polycarbophil (Fibercon®)**
   chewable tablets

Anti-motility Agents

Mechanism of Action: inhibits peristalsis and prolongs transit time
Side Effects: rash, <u>nausea</u>, <u>vomiting</u>, <u>constipation</u>, <u>abdominal cramps</u>, <u>dry mouth</u>, <u>abdominal distention</u>, <u>fatigue</u>

*Loperamide (Imodium®)**
tablet: 2 mg
capsule: 2 mg
liquid: 1 mg/5 ml

Diphenoxylate/atropine (Lomotil®)
solution: 2.5 mg/0.025 mg/5 ml
tablet: 2.5 mg/0.025 mg

Other Agents

Octreotide (Sandostatin®)
Mechanism of Action: mimics natural somatostatin and decreases gastric fluid
Indication: treatment of diarrhea secondary to chemotherapy that is refractory to other antidiarrheals
Side Effects: flushing, edema, fatigue, headache, <u>anorexia</u>, <u>nausea</u> and <u>vomiting</u>, increased liver function tests
injection: 0.05 mg/ml, 0.1 mg/ml, 0.5 mg/ml

Codeine
Mechanism of Action: unknown
Side Effects: constipation—incidence >10 %

Laxatives

Stool Softeners

Docusate (Colace®)**
many different salts
capsules or liquid

Stimulants

Side Effects: <u>abdominal cramping</u>

Senna (Sennokot)**
tablet

*Casanthranol **used in combination with
    docusate (Pericolace®)***
capsules or liquid

Nisacodyl (Dulcolax®)**
tablets
rectal solution
suppository

Bulk-forming Agents

Side Effects: <u>bowel obstruction</u>, <u>diarrhea</u>, <u>constipation</u>, <u>abdominal cramps</u>
Note: Give with adequate amounts of fluid and use cautiously in patients who cannot
        take adequate amounts of fluid or who are at risk for bowel obstruction

Psyllium (Metamucil®, Citrucel®, Perdiem®)**
granules
powder
chewable squares
wafers

Hyperosmotic Laxatives

Side Effects: headache, <u>vomiting</u>, dizziness, confusion, <u>diarrhea</u>

Glycerine**
oral solution
rectal solution and suppository

Mineral oil**
oral solution
rectal liquid

Saline Laxatives

Side Effects: dizziness, visual disturbances, dyspnea, <u>nausea</u>, <u>constipation</u>, <u>abdominal pain</u>,
        headache

Magnesium hydroxide (Milk of magnesia®)**
liquid, tablet

Magnesium citrate**
oral solution

Dibasic sodium phosphate (Fleet®)**
enema
oral solution

Table App B2   Anti-Diarrheals

Class	Drug	Route Powder	Route Other	Route Liquid	Mechanism of Action	Side Effects	Comments
Bulk-forming agent	Psyllium (Metamucil, Citrucel)	x	Chewable wafer	x	Absorbs water from intestine	EPS, sedation, hypotension	
	Calium polycarbophil (Fibercon)		Chewable wafer				Good first line agent
	Attapulgite (Kaopectate)		Chewable wafer	x			Good first line agent
Anti-motility agent	Loperaminde (Imodium)		Tablet capsule	x	Inhibits peristalsis Prolongs transit time	Rash, nausea, vomiting, dry mouth, abdominal cramps, constipation	Use caution if diarrhea may be infectious.
	Diphenoxylate/atropine (Lomotil)						
Miscellaneous anti-diarrheal	Octreotide (Sandostatin)		IV		Mimics somatato-statin drecreases fluid	Rash, flushing, edema, fatigue, headache, dizziness, increase LFT	Use as alternative to other therapy.

Key: IV = intravenous; LFT = Liver function tests

Table App B3   Laxatives

Class	Drug	Route Tablet	Route Capsule	Route Suppository	Route Other	Mechanism of Action	Side Effects	Comments
Stool softener	Docusate (Colace)		x		Liquid	Reduces surface tension of the stool to allow softening	Diarrhea, abdominal cramping	Available in many different salts
Stimulant	Senna (Sennokot)	x				Stimulates myenteric plexus	Abdominal cramping, diarrhea	
Stimulant	Bisacodyl (Dulcolax)	x		x	Rectal solution			
Bulk-forming agent	Psyllium (Metamucil, Citrucil, Perdium)	Granules, po chewable squares, chewable wafers				Holds water in stool	Abdominal cramping, diarrhea, constipation, bowel obstruction	May be used for diarrhea or constipation
Hyperosmotic laxative	Glycerine	Oral solution rectal solution		x		Local irritation	Headache, vomiting, dizziness, confusion, diarrhea	
Hyperosmotic laxative	Mineral oil	Oral solution rectal solution						
Saline laxative	Magnesium hydroxide (Milk of Magnesia)	x			Liquid	Retain water in intestinal lumen	Dizziness, visual disturbances, dyspnea, nausea, constipation	
Saline laxative	Dibasic sodium phosphate (Fleet)	x				Unkown	Mood changes, increased appetite, hypotension, tachycardia	Well tolerated in younger patients

Key: IV = intravenous; LFT = Liver function tests

Agents for Oral Care

Mouth care is important to prevent possible infection and/or irritation. Mucositis can be painful for patients and the use of topical anesthetic agents and healing agents may be beneficial. Oral candidiasis is common especially in patients receiving antibiotic therapy. There are many different products available; only a few are described below.

Cleansing Agents

Chlorhexidine (Peridex®)**
  mint flavor oral rinse (contains alcohol)

Healing/Coating Agents

Sucralfate (Carafate®)
Tannic acid (Zilactin Gel®)**

Topical Anesthetics

Benzocaine
Viscous lidocaine
Diclonine hydrochloride

Analgesic Agents (see Pain Medications below)

Mucositis Mouthwashes

These preparations are institution-specific, usually containing some combination of nystatin, Maalox®/Mylanta®, diphenhydramine, hydrocortisone, and tetracycline.

Antifungal Agents

Fluconazole (Diflucan®) tablets, suspension, injection
Nystatin (Mycostatin®) suspension
Clotrimazole (Mycelex®) troches
Used prophylactically or as treatment for oral candidiasis

Pain Medications

Pain can be caused by bone infiltration, nerve compression or infiltration, visceral involvement, and raised intracranial pressure. Other causes may be related to the therapy such as postoperative acute pain, postoperative neuralgia, phantom limb pain, and postradiation inflammation or fibrosis. Cancer may also cause constipation, bed sores, lymphedema or candidiasis which can be painful. The choice of agents used depends on the cause of pain. When patients complain of pain, decisions of therapy should be based on the severity of pain. The World Health Organization (WHO) has advocated a three-step analgesic ladder. See Figure App B1 for more details. Table App B4 describes drugs used for relief of mild to moderate pain and Table App B5 describes drugs used for relief of moderate to severe pain.

Table App B4   Drugs for Relief of Mild to Moderate Pain

Drug	Analgesic Class	Dosage Forms	Starting Dose	Max Daily	May Crush
Acetaminophen (Tylenol)	Miscellaneous	PO = 325 mg, 500 mg PR = 650 mg	650mg q 4-6 hrs prn	4000 mg	*
Choline Magnesium Trisalicylate (Trilisate)	NSAID	PO = 500 mg, 750 mg,1000 mg	500-1000 mg q 8-12 hrs	4000 mg	*
Codeine (Various)	Opioid narcotic	PO = 15 mg, 30 mg, 60 mg IM = 30 mg/mL	10-20 mg q 4-6 prn	360 mg	*
Codeine/Acetaminophen (Tylenol #3)	Opioid narcotic	PO = 30 mg codeine; 300 mg acetaminophen	1-2 tablets q 4-6 hrs prn	360 mg	*
Ibuprofen (Motrin, Advil)	NSAID	PO = 200 mg, 400 mg, 600 mg, 800 mg	400 mg q 4-6 hrs prn	3200 mg	*
Ketorolac (Toradol)	NSAID	PO = 10 mg IM/IV = 15 mg, 30 mg	10 mg q 6 hrs prn 5-30 mg IV/IM q 6 hrs prn	40 mg 120 mg	*
Naproxen (Naprosyn)	NSAID	PO = 250 mg, 500 mg	250 mg q 6-8 hrs prn	1500 mg	*
Propoxyphene (Darvon)	Opioid narcotic	PO = 65 mg	65 mg q 4-6 hrs prn	390 mg	
Propoxyphene/Acetaminophen (Darvocet N-100)	Opioid narcotic	PO = 100 mg propxyphene 650 mg acetaminophen	100 mg q 4-6 hrs prn	600 mg	
Salsalate (Disalcid)	NSAID	PO = 500 mg, 750 mg	1500 mg bid	3000 mg	*
Tramadol (Ultram)	Miscellaneous	PO = 50 mg	50 mg q 4-6 hrs	400 mg	*

Key: IM = Intramuscular; IV = Intravenous; NSAID = Non-Steroidal Anti-inflammatory Drug; PO = By mouth; PR = Per rectal

Table App B5   Drugs for Relief of Moderate to Severe Pain

Drug	Analgesic Class	Dosage Forms	Starting Dose	Duration	May Crush
Codeine/Acetaminophen (Tylenol #3)	Opioid narcotic	PO = 30 mg codeine; 325 mg acetaminophen	1-2 tablets q 4-6 hrs prn	3-6 hrs	
Fentanyl (Duragesic)	Opioid narcotic	TD = 25 mcg/hr, 50 mcg/hr, 75 mcg/hr, 100 mcg/hr	25 mcg/hr TD q 72 hrs	48-72 hrs	*
		IM = 50 mcg/mL	1-2 mcg/kg	1-2 hrs	
		IV = 50 mcg/mL	1-2 mcg/kg	0.5-1 hr	
Hydrocodone/Acetaminophen (Vicodin, Lortab)	Opioid narcotic	PO = 5 mg hydrocone; 500 mg Acetaminophen	1-2 tablets q 4-6 hrs prn	3-6 hrs	*
Hydromorphone (Dilaudid)	Opioid narcotic	PO = 1 mg, 2 mg, 3 mg, 4 mg, 8 mg	2 mg q 4-6 hrs prn	4-5 hrs	*
		IM = 1 mg/mL, 2 mg/mL	2 mg q 4-6 hrs prn	3-4 hrs	
		IV = 1 mg/mL, 2 mg/mL	2 mg q 4-6 hrs prn	3-4 hrs	
Morphine Sulfate (Various)	Opioid narcotic	PO = 10 mg, 15 mg, 30 mg	10-30 mg q 4 hrs prn	4-5 hrs	*
		IM = 0.5 mg/mL, 1 mg/mL, 2 mg/mL	2-10 mg q 4 hrs prn	4-5 hrs	
		IV = 0.5 mg/mL, 1 mg/mL, 2 mg/mL	2-10 mg q 4 hrs prn	4-5 hrs	
Morphine Sulfate Sustained Release (MS Contin, Kadian)	Opioid narcotic	PO (SR) = 15 mg, 30 mg, 60 mg, 100 mg, 200 mg	15-30 mg q 8-12 hrs prn	8-12 hrs	
Oxycodone (OxyIR)	Opioid narcotic	PO = 5 mg	5 mg q 6 hrs prn	4-5 hrs	*
Oxycodone Sustained Release (Ocycontin)	Opioid narcotic	PO = 10 mg, 20 mg, 40 mg, 70 mg	10 mg q 12 hrs	8-12 hrs	
Oxycodone/Acetaminophen (Tylox, Percocet)	Opioid narcotic	PO = 5 mg oxycodone; 325 mg acetaminophen (Percocet); 500 mg acetaminophen; (Tylox)	1-2 tablets q 4-6 hrs prn	3-6 hrs	*

Key: IM = Intramuscular; IV = Intravenous; PO = By mouth; TD = Transdermal; SR = Sustained Release

Non-Opioid Analgesics

Acetaminophen (Tylenol®)**
Mechanism of Action: inhibits the synthesis of prostaglandins
Indication: used as antipyretic and to treat mild to moderate pain; used mostly in combination with a narcotic analgesic
Side Effects: rash (rarely), <u>nausea</u> and <u>vomiting</u>
Dosage Forms: various liquid formulations (ask pharmacist for clarification of available forms)
tablet: 325 mg, 500 mg, 650 mg
caplet: 160 mg, 325 mg, 500 mg
suppository: 120mg, 125 mg, 300 mg, 325 mg, 650 mg

Non-Steroidal Anti-Inflammatory Drugs (NSAIDs)

Mechanism of Action: inhibits the synthesis of prostaglandins by decreasing the activity of the enzyme, cyclo-oxygenase
Indication: used as antipyretic, anti-inflammatory agent, and to treat mild to moderate pain before narcotics are tried
Side Effects: <u>gastric and duodenal ulcers</u>, rash, <u>abdominal cramps</u>, headache, fluid retention
Dosing: <u>Food may decrease absorption and decrease time to peak effect.</u>

Opioids

Mechanism of Action: bind to opiate receptors in the CNS, causing inhibition of ascending pain pathways, altering the perception of and response to pain
Indication: used to treat moderate to severe pain
Side Effects: sedation, decreased respiration, hypotension, weakness, <u>nausea and vomiting</u>, <u>constipation</u> (most commonly seen with codeine), <u>paralytic ileus</u>, decreased urination, pruritus

Hydromorphone (Dilaudid®)
injection: 1 mg/ml, 2 mg/ml, 3 mg/ml, 4 mg/ml,10 mg/ml
tablets: 2 mg, 4 mg
suppository: 3 mg

Fentanyl
transdermal patch: (Duragesic®) 25 mcg/hr, 50 mcg/hr, 75 mcg/hr, 100 mcg/hr
injection: 0.05 mg/ml
lozenge: (Oralet®) 200 mcg, 300 mcg, 400 mcg

Morphine (MS Contin®, MS IR®, Kadian®)
regular release tablets: 15 mg, 30 mg
sustained release tablets: 15 mg, 30 mg, 60 mg, 100 mg
oral solution: 10 mg/5 ml, 20 mg/5 ml
suppository: 5 mg, 10 mg, 20 mg, 30 mg
injection: 1 mg/ml, 2 mg/ml, 5 mg/ml, 10 mg/ml, 15 mg/ml

Oxycodone (Oxycotin®)
regular release tablets: 5 mg
sustained release tablets: 10 mg, 20 mg, 40 mg

Combination products:
Hydrocodone and acetaminophen (Lorcet®, Lortab®,Vicodin®)
Oxycodone and acetaminophen (Roxicodone®, Percocet®,Tylox®)
Oxycodone and aspirin (Percodan®)
Codeine and acetaminophen (Tylenol #3®)
Propoxyphene and acetaminophen (Darvocet-N-100®)
Propoxyphene (Darvon®)

Miscellaneous Agents

There are times when oncology patients require supportive therapy with medications. Therapies can cause xerostomia requiring saliva stimulants or artificial saliva. Anorexia may also be a problem for numerous reasons and megestrol or dronabinol may help to stimulate appetite. Whenever pancreatic malabsorption occurs, pancreatic enzymes may be indicated. While antibiotics are not here discussed in detail, it should be noted that they can cause multiple nutritional side effects such as <u>diarrhea</u>, <u>nausea</u>, and oral candidiasis.

Saliva Stimulant

Pilocarpine (Salagen®)
Mechanism of action: stimulates cholinergic receptors in the mouth to produce saliva
Dose: 5 mg tablet three times a day

Appetite Stimulant

Megestrol (Megace®)
Dose: 800mg daily, available in 20 mg/ml suspension
Side Effects: edema, breakthrough bleeding and amenorrhea, headache, rash, <u>weight gain</u>

Dronabinol (Marinol®)
Dose: 2.5 mg tablet twice a day
Side Effects: mood changes, <u>increased appetite</u>, hypotension, tachycardia, blurred vision

Metoclopramide (Reglan®)
Cisapride (Propulsid®)
Dose: 10 mg tablet four times a day
Side Effects: weakness, restlessness, drowsiness, <u>diarrhea</u>, insomnia, rash, <u>dry mouth</u>, extrapyramidal reactions (rare)

Pancreatic Enzymes

(See Table App B6 for a list of available agents)
Side Effects: <u>nausea</u>, <u>abdominal cramps</u>, <u>constipation</u>, <u>diarrhea</u>

Figure App B1   Three-Step Analgesic Ladder

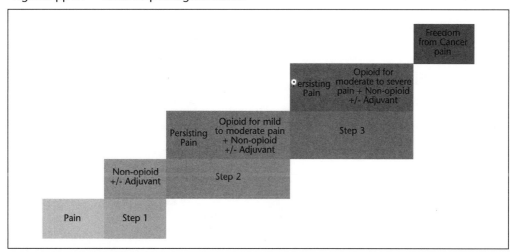

Adapted from *Clinical Practice Guidelines: Management of Cancer Pain:* Clinical Practice Guideline Number 9.

Table App B6   Pancreatic Enzyme Preparations

Product	Dosage Form	Do Not Crush	Lipase USP Units	Amylase USP Units	Protease USP Units
Cotazym® Ku-Syme® HP	Capsule		8000	30,000	30,000
Cotazym®-S	Capsule, enteric coated microspheres	*	5000	20,000	20,000
Creon®	Enteric coated microspheres	*	8000	30,000	13,000
Entolase® Pancrease® Protilase®	Capsule, delayed release	*	4000	20,000	25,000
Entolase HP®	Enteric coated microbeads	*	8000	40,000	50,000
Festal® II	Tablet, delayed release	*	6000	30,000	20,000
Ilozyme®	Tablet		11,000	30,000	30,000
Pancrease® MT	Tablet				
4	Capsule, enteric coated microtablets	*	40,000	12,000	12,000
10		*	10,000	30,000	30,000
16		*	16,000	48,000	48,000
Viokase®	Powder		16,800 per 0.7 g	70,000 per 0.7 g	70,000 per 0.7 g
	Tablet		8000	30,000	30,000
Zymase®	Capsule, enteric coated spheres	*	12,000	24,000	24,000

Note: When crushing, please consult a pharmacist for clarification.

Drug Manufacturers

Actigall®
    Summit; Fort Lee, NJ
Anzemet®
    Aventis; Kansas City, MO
Ativan®
    Wyeth-Ayerst; Philadelphia, PA
Carafate®
    Aventis; Kansas City, MO
Citrucel®
    SmithKline Beecham; Philadelphia, PA
Colace®
    Roberts; Eatontown, NJ
Compazine®
    SmithKline Beecham; Philadelphia, PA
Cotazym®
    Organon; West Orange, NJ
Creon®
    Solvay; Marietta, GA
Darvocet-N-100®
    Lilly; Indianapolis, IN
Darvon®
    Lilly; Indianapolis, IN
Decadron®
    Merck; West Point, PA

Diazepam®
    Roche; Nutley, NJ
Diflucan®
    Pfizer; New York, NY
Dilaudid®
    Knoll Labs; Mt. Olive, NJ
Droperidol®
    Astra; Wayne, PA
Dulcolax®
    Novartis; Summit, NJ
Duragesic®
    Janssen; Titusville, NJ
FiberCon®
    Lederle; Pearl River, NJ
Fleet®
    Fleet; Lynchburg, VA
Haldol®
    Ortho-McNeil; Fort Washington, PA
Ilozyme®
    Adria; Kalamazoo, MI
Imodium®
    Janssen; Titusville, NJ
Imuran®
    GlaxoWellcome; Triangle Park, NJ

Kadian®
    Faulding; Elizabeth, NJ
Kaopectate®
    Upjohn; Kalamazoo, MI
Ku-Zyme®
    Schwarz Pharma; Mequon, WI
Kytril®
    SmithKline Beecham; Philadelphia, PA
Lomotil®
    Searle; Chicago, IL
Lorcet®
    Forest; St. Louis, MO
Lortab®
    UCB Pharma; Symrna, GA
Marinol®
    Roxane; Columbus, OH
Megace®
    Bristol Myers Squibb; Princeton, NJ
Metamucil®
    Proctor & Gamble; Cincinnati, OH
Milk of Magnesia®
    Glenwood; Tenafly, NJ
MS Contin®
    Purdue Frederick; Norwalk, CT
MS IR®
    Prudue Frederick; Norwalk, CT
Mycelex®
    Alza; Palo Alto, CA
Mycostatin®
    Lederle; Pearl River, NY
Octreotide®
    Novartis; Summit, NJ
Oralet®
    Abbott; Abbott Park, IL
Oxycotin®
    Purdue Frederick; Norwalk, CT
Pancrease®
    Ortho-McNeil; Fort Washington, PA
Percocet®
    Endo Labs; Chadds Ford, PA
Percodan®
    Endo Labs; Chadds Ford, PA
Peri-Colace®
    Roberts; Eatontown, NJ

Peridex®
    Proctor & Gamble; Cincinnati, OH
Phenergan®
    Wyeth-Ayerst; Philadelphia, PA
Prograf®
    Fujisawa USA; Deerfield, IL
Propulsid®
    Janssen; Titusville, NJ
Protilase®
    Rugby; Corona, CA
Rapamune®
    Wyeth-Ayerst; St. David's, PA
Reglan®
    A. H. Robins; Philadelphia, PA
Roxicodone®
    Roxane; Columbus, OH
Salagen®
    MGI; Minnetonka, MN
Senokot®
    Purdue Frederick; Norwalk, CT
Torecan®
    Roxane; Columbus, OH
Trans Derm®
    Novartis; Summit, NJ
Trilafon®
    Schering; Kenilworth, NJ
Tylenol®
    Ortho McNeil; Fort Washington, PA
Tylenol #3®
    Ortho-McNeil; Fort Washington, PA
Tylox®
    Ortho-McNeil; Fort Washington, PA
Vicodin®
    Knoll Labs; Mt. Olive, NJ
Viokase®
    A. H. Robins; Philadelphia, PA
Zilactin Gel®
    Zila; Phoeniz, PA
Zofran®
    Glaxo-Wellcome; RTP, NC
Zymase®
    Oragnon, West Orange, NJ

Sources

Lacy C. Armstrong LL, Ingrim N, Lance LL. *Drug Information Handbook.* 1997-98. Hudson, Ohio: Lexi-Comp Inc; 1997.

McEvoy GK, editor. *AHFS: Drug Information.* Bethesda, Md: American Society of Health-System Pharmacists; 1997.

Clinical Practice Guidelines: Management of Cancer Pain. US Department of Health and Human Services. Agency for Health Care Policy and Research. Rockville, Md AHCPR Publication No. 94-0592. March 1994.

Appendix C

Resources

Laura Elliot, RD   Dee Grabbard, RD

For the Professional
Publications

Cancer
An interdisciplinary international journal of the American Cancer Society. $315/yr - 30 issues. 800/511-3989.

CA-A Cancer Journal For Clinicians (ACS)
For a free subscription, contact your local ACS chapter.

Cancer Practice (ACS)
A bimonthly multidisciplinary journal of cancer care. $39/yr 800/777-2295.

Cancer Prevention International
A quarterly journal published by the Society for Nutritional Oncology Adjuvant Therapy. Included with membership to NOAT. $75 for allied health professionals. 847/342-6484.

Environmental Nutrition Newsletter
A monthly newsletter including alternative therapy, research and consumer topics. $30/yr - 12 issues. 800/829-5384.

Journal of Clinical Oncology
Official journal of the Society of Clinical Oncology. $201/yr W.B. Saunders 407/345-2500.

Nutrition in Complementary Care
A quarterly newsletter of the Nutrition in Complementary Care Dietetics Practice Group of the American Dietetic Association. Contact the American Dietetic Association at 800/877-1600 for current administrative editor.

Oncology
A monthly journal with articles pertaining to the practical management of cancer patients. $85/yr. PRR, Inc. 516/424-8900.

Oncology Nursing Forum.
The official journal of Oncology Nursing Society which conveys developments in practice, technology and research to promote quality care. $71/year - 10 issues. Oncology Nursing Press, Inc. 412/921-7373.

ON-LINE
A quarterly publication by the Oncology Nutrition Dietetic Practice Group (ONDPG) of the ADA available to ONDPG non-members. Contact ADA at 800/877-1600 for subscription information.

Books

Berger AM. *Principles and Practice of Supportive Oncology.* Lippincott-Raven Press; 1998. Integrates the elements of palliative care; authored by members of the interdisciplinary professional oncology team. Includes chapters on nutritional support, hydration, survivorship, medical ethics, and quality of life.

Bloch AS. ed. *Nutrition Management of the Cancer Patient.* Aspen Publishers, 1990. An in-depth nutrition and cancer resource with chapters on specific patient populations and methods of management.

Cooper GM. *Elements of Human Cancer*, Jones and Bartlett Publishers; 1992. An overview of cancer, treatment, staging and causes including dietary factors and diet in cancer prevention.

DeVita VT, Hellman S, and Rosenberg SA. *Cancer Principles and Practice of Oncology*. J. B. Lippincott Co. 1989. An in-depth review of research on diet and carcinogenesis including clinical trials and the physician as a promoter of diet.

Gallagher-Allred CR. *Nutritional Care of the Terminally Ill*, Aspen Publications; 1989. A guide to nutrition in palliative care including symptom management, the role of the dietitian on the care team, ethnic beliefs about food and dying, and implementation and evaluation of practice guidelines.

Greenwald P, Kramer BS, and Weed D. *Cancer Prevention and Control*. Marcel Dekker, Inc, 1995. A reference on cancer prevention containing information on specific cancer risks and attributed causal factors.

Groeger JS. *Critical Care of the Cancer Patient*. Mosby-Year Book, Inc., 1991. A reference showing the effects of system failure, gastrointestinal and neurologic toxicity and briefly, nutrition support.

Holland J et al. *Cancer Medicine*. Fourth Edition, Vol. 1 and 2, Lea and Febiger Publishers, 1997. An in-depth resource on medical oncology with a chapter on diet, chemoprevention, and cancer.

Holland J, ed. *Psyco-Oncology*, Oxford University Press, 1998. A textbook written by interdisciplinary professionals describing the psychological and behavioral risk factors in cancer and their interventions. It also includes psychological issues related to cancer sites, alternative and complementary therapies and palliative care. Each section includes extensive references.

Ramstack JL, Rosenbaum EH. *Nutrition for the Chemotherapy Patient*, Bull Publishing Co, 1990. A guide to nutrition therapy during chemotherapy for patients and professionals.

Media

A Diet Nutrition and Cancer Video. Health Science Institute, 1350 Beverly Rd., Suite 115-206, McLean Va. 22101. 800/474-6211. A 45 minute program about carcinogenesis, nutrients in prevention and promotion, dietary guidelines, and nutritional care of patients. A 15-minute video on phytochemicals is also available.

Medical Nutrition Therapy Across the Continuum of Care, 2nd ed. 1997. The American Dietetic Association and Morrison Health Care, Inc. 800/877-1600 ext. 5000. Protocols, forms, videotapes, and disks designed to help professionals communicate the benefits of medical nutrition therapy. Sections specific to medical oncology and radiation oncology included.

Patient-Generated Subjective Global Assessment video. American Dietetic Association, 800/877-1600 ext. 5000. A video produced by the Oncology Nutrition Dietetic Practice Group of the American Dietetic Association, covering the patient-generated subjective global assessment.

Walker M., Masino K. *Oncology Nutrition: Patient Education Materials*. 1998. Chicago, Ill. 800/877-1600, ext. 4814. A packet of education materials developed by the Oncology Nutrition Dietetic Practice Group of the American Dietetic Association designed to help the dietetics professional ease the symptoms and side effects of cancer and its treatment. Contains 18 reproducible patient education sheets.

For the Patient
Publications

Eating Hints—Recipes and Tips for Better Nutrition During Treatment. National Cancer Institute, NIH Publication No. 98-2079, rev. 1998. This patient guide offers modified diets, tips for managing side effects, and recipes included for those undergoing treatment. Contact 800/4-CANCER for a publication catalog and a free copy.

Feeling Good: Nutritional Planning to Improve Your Cancer Therapy. Abby Bloch, MS, RD. Free from Mead Johnson Nutritionals; for a copy contact your local sales representative. This patient guide includes tips for managing side effects and a limited list of the calorie content of foods.

Nutrition: An Ally in Cancer Therapy. Free from Ross Medical Nutritional System; contact your local sales representative. An easy-to-read brief overview of common nutrition problems in cancer therapy, and recipes using Ross products.

Nutrition for Patients Receiving Chemotherapy and Radiation Treatment, by the American Cancer Society. For more information call 800/ACS-2345. A patient guide of common nutrition problems in cancer therapy. Also available are brochures, videos, posters, and programs consistent with the 1996 Dietary Guidelines for Americans, available free for general health promotion.

Books

Dodd MJ. *Managing the Side Effects of Chemotherapy and Radiation Therapy.* Prentice Hall Press; 1996. A guide for cancer patients and their families that includes descriptions, expected duration, and self care measures for nutritional problems encountered during treatments.

Weihofen, D *The Cancer Survival Cookbook.* Chronimed Publishing. $14.95 800/848-2793. A patient friendly book written by a dietitian with 200 quick and easy recipes and helpful eating hints.

Media

Farmer G. *Pass the Calories, Please!* American Dietetic Association; 1994. 800/877-1600. A free video for patient education reviewing the importance of eating well during treatment, with tips on improving intake.

Fighting Back with Nutrition, Bristol-Meyers Squibb Oncology/Immunology, Princeton, NJ 08543, or contact your Mead-Johnson representative. A free video for patient education. The video reviews the importance of eating well during treatment, with tips on improving intake.

Nutrition for Prevention, Adjuvant Therapy of Cancer. Food Safety Health Science Institute. Each 15 minute video targets lay people.

Taking Charge...Nutrition for Cancer Patients, Available from your Ross Laboratories representative. A 22-minute videotape that explains the importance of nutrition. It includes nutritional tips and hints to help cancer patients eat well.

On-line

Agencies and Organizations

American Cancer Society (ACS)
1599 Clifton Road, NE
Atlanta, GA 30329-4251
800/ACS-2345
Local chapters are listed in white pages of the
telephone book.

The American Dietetic Association (ADA)
Consumer Nutrition Hotline
216 W. Jackson Boulevard
Chicago, IL 60606-6995
800/366-1655

American Institute for Cancer Research (AICR)
1759 R Street NW,
Washington DC. 20009
800/843-8114 (Nutrition Hotline)
202/328-7744

National Association of Home Care
Directory of local hospices
202/547-7424

National Cancer Institute (NCI)
9000 Rockville Pike, Bldg 31, Room 10A07
Bethesda, MD 20892
301/496-8664 (Consumer Information) or
800/4-CANCER
A cancer information service through the
U.S. government.

United Ostomy Association
36 Executive Park, Suite 120
Irvine, CA 36714
714/660-8624

Index

Tables & Worksheets for PG-SGA Scoring

The PG-SGA numerical score is derived by totaling the scores from boxes A-D of the PG-SGA on the reverse side. Boxes 1-4 are designed to be completed by the patient. The points assigned to items in boxes 1-4 are noted parenthetically after each item. The following worksheets are offered as aids for calcuating scores of sections that are not so marked.

Table 1 - Scoring Weight (wt) Loss

Determined by adding points for subacute and acute wt change. **Subacute:** If information is available about weight loss during past 1 month, add the point score to the points for acute wt change. Only include the wt loss over 6 months if the wt from 1 month is unavailable. **Acute:** refers to wt change during past two weeks. Add 1 point to subacute score if patient lost wt; add no points if patient gained or maintained wt during the past two weeks.

Wt loss in 1 month	Points	Wt loss in 6 months
10% or greater	4	20% or greater
5-9.9%	3	10 -19.9%
3-4.9%	2	6 - 9.9%
2-2.9%	1	2 - 5.9%
0-1.9%	0	0 - 1.9%

Points for Box 1 = Subacute + Acute = [ ] A

Table 2 - Scoring criteria for disease &/or condition

Score is derived by adding 1 point for each of the conditions listed below that pertain to the patient.

Category	Points
Cancer	1
AIDS	1
Pulmonary or cardiac cachexia	1
Presence of decubitus, open wound, or fistula	1
Presence of trauma	1
Age greater than 65 years	1

Points for Box 2 = [ ] B

Table 3 Worksheet. Scoring Metabolic Stress

Score for metabolic stress is determined by a number of variables known to increase protein & calorie needs. The score is additive so that a patient who has a fever of > 102 degrees (3 points) and is on 10 mg of prednisone chronically (2 points) would have an additive score for this section of 5 points.

Stress	none (0)	low (1)	moderate (2)	high (3)
Fever	no fever	>99 and <101	≥101 and <102	≥102
Fever duration	no fever	<72 hrs	72 hrs	> 72 hrs
Steroids	no steroids	low dose (<10mg prednisone equivalents/day)	moderate dose (≥10 and <30mg prednisone equivalents/day)	high dose steroids (≥30mg prednisone equivalents/day)

Points for Table 3 = [ ] C

Table 4 Worksheet - Physical Examination

Physical exam includes a subjective evaluation of 3 aspects of body composition: fat, muscle, & fluid status. Since this is subjective, each aspect of the exam is rated for degree of deficit. Definition of categories: 0 = no deficit, 1+ = mild deficit, 2+ = moderate deficit, 3+ = severe deficit. Degree of muscle deficit takes precedence over fat deficit. Rating of deficit in these categories are *not* additive but a used to clinically assess the degree of deficit (or presence of excess fluid).

Fat Stores:

orbital fat pads	0	1+	2+	3+
triceps skin fold	0	1+	2+	3+
fat overlying lower ribs	0	1+	2+	3+
Global fat deficit rating	**0**	**1+**	**2+**	**3+**

Fluid Status:

ankle edema	0	1+	2+	3+
sacral edema	0	1+	2+	3+
ascites	0	1+	2+	3+
Global fluid status rating	**0**	**1+**	**2+**	**3+**

Muscle Status:

temples (temporalis muscle)	0	1+	2+	3+
clavicles (pectoralis & deltoids)	0	1+	2+	3+
shoulders (deltoids)	0	1+	2+	3+
interosseous muscles	0	1+	2+	3+
scapula (latissimus dorsi, trapezius, deltoids)	0	1+	2+	3+
thigh (quadriceps)	0	1+	2+	3+
calf (gastrocnemius)	0	1+	2+	3+
Global muscle status rating	**0**	**1+**	**2+**	**3+**

Point score for the physical exam is determined by the overall subjective rating of total body deficit; again muscle deficit takes precedence over fat loss or fluid excess.

No deficit	score = 0 points
Mild deficit	score = 1 point
Moderate deficit	score = 2 points
Severe deficit	score = 3 points

Points for Worksheet 4 = [ ] D

Table 5 Worksheet PG-SGA Global Assessment Categories

	Stage A	Stage B	Stage C
Category	Well-nourished	Moderately malnourished or suspected malnutrition	Severely malnourished
Weight	No wt loss **or** Recent non-fluid wt gain	~5% wt loss within 1 month (or 10% in 6 months) No wt stabilization or wt gain (i.e., continued wt loss)	a. > 5% loss in 1 month (or >10% loss in 6 months) b. No wt stabilization or wt gain (i.e., continued wt loss)
Nutrient Intake	No deficit **or** Significant recent improvement	Definite decrease in intake	Severe deficit in intake
Nutrition Impact Symptoms	None **or** Significant recent improvement allowing adequate intake	Presence of nutrition impact symptoms (Box 3 of PG-SGA)	Presence of nutrition impact symptoms (Box 3 of PG-SGA)
Functioning	No deficit **or** Significant recent improvement	Moderate functional deficit **or** Recent deterioration	Severe functional deficit **or** recent significant deterioration
Physical Exam	No deficit **or** Chronic deficit but with recent clinical improvement	Evidence of mild to moderate loss of SQ fat &/or muscle mass &/or muscle tone on palpation	Obvious signs of malnutrition (e.g., severe loss of SQ tissues, possible edema)

Global PG-SGA rating (A, B, or C) = [ ]

Scored Patient-Generated Subjective Global Assessment (PG-SGA)

Patient ID Information

History

1. Weight *(See Table 1 Worksheet)*

In summary of my current and recent weight:

I currently weigh about _____ pounds
I am about _____ feet _____ tall

One months ago I weighed about _____ pounds
Six months ago I weighed about _____ pounds

During the past two weeks my weight has:

☐ decreased (1) ☐ not changed (0) ☐ increased (0)

[ ]

2. Food Intake: As compared to my normal, I would rate my food intake during the past month as:

☐ unchanged (0)
☐ more than usual
☐ less than usual (1)

I am now taki*ng:*

☐ *normal food* but less than normal (1)
☐ little solid food (2)
☐ only liquids (3)
☐ only nutritonal supplements (3)
☐ very little of anything (4)
☐ only tube feedings or only nutrition by vein

[ ]

3. Symptoms: I have had the following problems that have kept me from eating enough during the past two weeks (check all that apply):

☐ no problems eating (0)

☐ no appetite, just did not feel like eating (3)

☐ nausea (1)   ☐ vomiting (3)
☐ constipation (1)   ☐ diarrhea (3)
☐ mouth sores (2)   ☐ dry mouth (1)
☐ things taste funny or have no taste (1) ☐ smells bother me (1)
☐ problems swallowing (2)   ☐ feel full quickly (1)
☐ pain; where? (3) _____
☐ other** (1) _____

** Examples: depression, money, or dental problems

[ ]

4. Activities and Function: Over the past month, I would generally rate my activity as:

☐ normal with no limitations (0)

☐ not my normal self, but able to be up and about with fairly normal activities (1)

☐ not feeling up to most things, but in bed less than half the day (2)

☐ able to do little activity and spend most of the day in bed or chair (3)

[ ]

Additive Score of the Boxes 1-4 [ ] **A**

The remainder of this form will be complete by your doctor, nurse, or therapist. Thank you.

5. Disease and its relation to nutritional requirements *(See Table 2)*

All relevant diagnoses (specify) _____

Primary disease stage (circle if known or appropriate)   I   II   III   IV   Other _____

Age _____

Numerical score from Table 2 [ ] **B**

6. Metabolic Demand *(See Table 3 Worksheet)*

☐ no stress   ☐ low stress   ☐ moderate stress   ☐ high stress

Numerical score from Table 3 [ ] **C**

7. Physical *(See Table 4 Worksheet)*

Numerical score from Table 4 [ ] **D**

Global Assessment *(See Table 5 Worksheet)*

☐ Well-nourished or anabolic (SGA-A)
☐ Moderate or suspected malnutrition (SGA-B)
☐ Severely malnourished (SGA-C)

Total numerical score of boxes A+B+C+D [ ]
(See triage recommendations below)

Clinician Signature _____ RD RN PA MD DO Other ___   Date _____

Nutritional Triage Recommendations: Additive score is used to define specific nutritional interventions including patient & family education, symptom management including pharmacologic intervention, and appropriate nutrient intervention (food, nutritional supplements, enteral, or parenteral triage). First line nutrition intervention includes optimal symptom management.

0-1	No intervention required at this time. Re-assessment on routine and regular basis during treatment.
2-3	Patient & family education by dietitian, nurse, or other clinician with pharmacologic intervention as indicated by symptom survey (Box 3) and laboratory values as appropriate.
4-8	Requires intervention by dietitian, in conjunction with nurse or physician, as indicated by symptoms survey (Box 3).
≥ 9	Indicates a critical need for improved symptom management and/or nutrient intervention options.